Nutrition in the Practice of Medicine: A Practical Approach

Editor

DAVID S. SERES

MEDICAL CLINICS OF NORTH AMERICA

www.medical.theclinics.com

Consulting Editor
JACK ENDE

September 2022 • Volume 106 • Number 5

ELSEVIER

1600 John F. Kennedy Boulevard • Suite 1800 • Philadelphia, Pennsylvania, 19103-2899

http://www.theclinics.com

MEDICAL CLINICS OF NORTH AMERICA Volume 106, Number 5
September 2022 ISSN 0025-7125, ISBN-13: 978-0-323-96183-7

Editor: Taylor Hayes
Developmental Editor: Arlene Campos

Medical Clinics of North America (ISSN 0025-7125) is published bimonthly by Elsevier Inc., 360 Park Avenue South, New York, NY 10010-1710. Months of publication are January, March, May, July, September, and November. Business and editorial offices: 1600 John F. Kennedy Boulevard, Suite 1800, Philadelphia, PA 19103-2899. Periodicals postage paid at New York, NY, and additional mailing offices. Subscription prices are USD $316.00 per year (US individuals), $956.00 per year (US institutions), $100.00 per year (US Students), $396.00 per year (Canadian individuals), $1,004.00 per year (Canadian institutions), $200.00 per year for (foreign students), $100.00 per year for (Canadian students), $439.00 per year (foreign individuals), and $1,004.00 per year (foreign institutions). To receive student/resident rate, orders must be accompanied by name of affiliated institution, date of term, and the signature of program/residency coordinator on institution letterhead. Orders will be billed at individual rate until proof of status is received. Foreign air speed delivery is included in all Clinics' subscription prices. All prices are subject to change without notice. **POSTMASTER:** Send address changes to *Medical Clinics of North America*, Elsevier Health Sciences Division, Subscription Customer Service, 3251 Riverport Lane, Maryland Heights, MO 63043. **Customer Service: Telephone: 1-800-654-2452** (U.S. and Canada); **1-314-447-8871** (outside U.S. and Canada). **Fax:** 314-447-8029. **E-mail: journalscustomerserviceusa@elsevier.com** (for print support); **journalsonlinesupport-usa@elsevier.com** (for online support).

Reprints. For copies of 100 or more of articles in this publication, please contact the Commercial Reprints Department, Elsevier Inc., 360 Park Avenue South, New York, NY 10010-1710. Tel.: 212-633-3874; Fax: 212-633-3820; E-mail: reprints@elsevier.com.

Medical Clinics of North America is also published in Spanish by McGraw-Hill Interamericana Editores S. A., P.O. Box 5-237, 06500 Mexico, D.F., Mexico.

Medical Clinics of North America is covered in *MEDLINE/PubMed (Index Medicus), Current Contents, ASCA, Excerpta Medica, Science Citation Index, and ISI/BIOMED.*

PROGRAM OBJECTIVE
The goal of the *Medical Clinics of North America* is to keep practicing physicians up to date with current clinical practice by providing timely articles reviewing the state of the art in patient care.

TARGET AUDIENCE
All practicing physicians and other healthcare professionals.

LEARNING OBJECTIVES
Upon completion of this activity, participants will be able to:
1. Review the risks and contributing factors of chronic disease and dietary nutrition disorders.
2. Explain the role of health care providers in nutritional management in promoting adherence to a balanced diet to reduce the risk of chronic disease and poor health outcomes.
3. Discuss strategies for promoting changes in dietary behaviors and nutritional adherence, such as the use of screening and assessment tools, cognitive behavioral therapy and motivational interviewing, medical treatments, and patient-centered collaborative care.

ACCREDITATION
The Elsevier Office of Continuing Medical Education (EOCME) is accredited by the Accreditation Council for Continuing Medical Education (ACCME) to provide continuing medical education for physicians.

The EOCME designates this journal-based CME activity for a maximum of 12 *AMA PRA Category 1 Credit(s)*™. Physicians should claim only the credit commensurate with the extent of their participation in the activity.

All other healthcare professionals requesting continuing education credit for this enduring material will be issued a certificate of participation.

DISCLOSURE OF CONFLICTS OF INTEREST
The EOCME assesses conflict of interest with its instructors, faculty, planners, and other individuals who are in a position to control the content of CME activities. All relevant conflicts of interest that are identified are thoroughly vetted by EOCME for fair balance, scientific objectivity, and patient care recommendations. EOCME is committed to providing its learners with CME activities that promote improvements or quality in healthcare and not a specific proprietary business or a commercial interest.

The planning committee, staff, authors and editors listed below have identified no financial relationships or relationships to products or devices they or their spouse/life partner have with commercial interest related to the content of this CME activity:
Alice S. Ammerman, DrPH; Adrianne Bendich, PhD, FASN; Sarah L. Booth, PhD; Gina Campanella, BS, RD, CDN; Tsz-Kiu Chui, MS, RD; Julianne G. Clina, MS; Julie Devinsky, RD; Gina Difusco, BS, RD, CDN; Sarah E. Ehrlicher, PhD, RD; Katie Ellison, MS, RD; David B. Gaviria, MPH, RD; Caitlin A. Hildebrand, MD, MPH; Daniela Jodorkovsky, MD; Thomas C. Keyserling, MD, MPH; Judith Korner, MD, PhD; Penny M. Kris-Etherton, PhD, RD, FAHA, FNLA, FASN, CLS; Nicole Kuerzi, BS, RD, CDN, CNSC; Walt Larimore, MD; Jim Mann, MD, PhD; Elizabeth Miracle, MS, RD, CSO, CDN, CNSC; Wasay A. Mohajir; Dónal O'Mathúna, PhD; Stephen J. O'Keefe, MD, PhD; Merlin Packiam; Alexander Panda, MD, PhD, MPH; Kristina Petersen, PhD, APD, FAHA; Sydney Pomenti, MD; Tirissa J. Reid, MD; Andrew Reynolds, PhD; Connie J. Rogers, Phd, MPH; Carmen D. Samuel-Hodge, RD, PhD; R. Drew Sayer, PhD Chinara Tate, PhD, RD; Doreen Thomas-Payne, MSN, BSN, RN, PMHNP-BC; Melissa Townsend, MS, RD, CDN; Ted Wilson, PhD

The planning committee, staff, authors, and editors listed below have identified financial relationships or relationships to products or devices they or their spouse/life partner have with commercial interest related to the content of this CME activity:
Michelle Christensen, MS, RD, CNSC: Employee: Coram LLC

David S. Seres, MD, ScM, PNS, FASPEN: Consultant: Community Surgical Supply, Fresenius Kabi USA, LLC

UNAPPROVED/OFF-LABEL USE DISCLOSURE
The EOCME requires CME faculty to disclose to the participants;
1. When products or procedures being discussed are off-label, unlabelled, experimental, and/or investigational (not US Food and Drug Administration [FDA] approved); and
2. Any limitations on the information presented, such as data that are preliminary or that represent ongoing research, interim analyses, and/or unsupported opinions. Faculty may discuss information about

pharmaceutical agents that is outside of FDA-approved labelling. This information is intended solely for CME and is not intended to promote off-label use of these medications. If you have any questions, contact the medical affairs department of the manufacturer for the most recent prescribing information.

TO ENROLL
To enroll in the *Medical Clinics of North America* Continuing Medical Education program, call customer service at 1-800-654-2452 or sign up online at http://www.theclinics.com/home/cme. The CME program is available to subscribers for an additional annual fee of USD 324.00.

METHOD OF PARTICIPATION
In order to claim credit, participants must complete the following;
1. Complete enrolment as indicated above.
2. Read the activity.
3. Complete the CME Test and Evaluation. Participants must achieve a score of 70% on the test. All CME Tests and Evaluations must be completed online.

CME INQUIRIES/SPECIAL NEEDS
For all CME inquiries or special needs, please contact elsevierCME@elsevier.com.

MEDICAL CLINICS OF NORTH AMERICA

FORTHCOMING ISSUES

November 2022
Clinical Psychiatry
Leo Sher, *Editor*

January 2023
Pulmonary Diseases
Daniel M. Goodenberger, *Editor*

March 2023
Women's Health
Melissa McNeil, *Editor*

RECENT ISSUES

July 2022
Communication Skills and Challenges in Medical Practice
Heather Hofmann, *Editor*

May 2022
Disease-Based Physical Examination
Paul Aronowitz, *Editor*

March 2022
Update in Preventive Cardiology
Douglas S. Jacoby, *Editor*

MEDICAL CLINICS OF NORTH AMERICA

CONTRIBUTORS

Contributors

CONSULTING EDITOR

JACK ENDE, MD, MACP
The Schaeffer Professor of Medicine, Perelman School of Medicine, University of Pennsylvania, Philadelphia, Pennsylvania, USA

EDITOR

DAVID S. SERES, MD, ScM, PNS, FASPEN
Professor of Medicine, Institute of Human Nutrition, Director of Medical Nutrition, Associate Clinical Ethicist, Columbia University Irving Medical Center, New York, New York, USA

AUTHORS

ALICE S. AMMERMAN, DrPH
Center for Health Promotion and Disease Prevention, Department of Nutrition, Gillings School of Global Public Health, The University of North Carolina at Chapel Hill, Chapel Hill, North Carolina, USA

ADRIANNE BENDICH, PhD, FASN
Nutrition and Health Book Series Editor, Springer/Nature, Wellington, Florida, USA

SARAH L. BOOTH, PhD
Senior Scientist, Jean Mayer USDA Human Nutrition Research Center on Aging, Tufts University, Boston, Massachusetts, USA

MICHELLE CHRISTENSEN, MS, RD, CDN, CNSC
Coram CVS Specialty Infusion Services (Coram)

TSZ-KIU CHUI, MS, RD
PhD Student, Department of Nutrition Sciences, The University of Alabama at Birmingham, Birmingham, Alabama, USA

JULIANNE G. CLINA, MS
PhD Student, Department of Nutrition Sciences, The University of Alabama at Birmingham, Birmingham, Alabama, USA

JULIE DEVINSKY, RD
Division of Digestive and Liver Diseases, Columbia University Irving Medical Center, New York, New York, USA

GINA DIFUSCO, BS, RD, CDN
Department of Food and Nutrition, NewYork-Presbyterian Hospital, Columbia University Irving Medical Center, New York, New York, USA

SARAH E. EHRLICHER, PhD, RD
Postdoctoral Fellow, Department of Nutrition Sciences, The University of Alabama at Birmingham, Birmingham, Alabama, USA

KATIE M. ELLISON, MS, RD
PhD Student, Department of Nutrition Sciences, The University of Alabama at Birmingham, Birmingham, Alabama, USA

DAVID B. GAVIRIA, MPH, RD
Center for Health Promotion and Disease Prevention, Department of Nutrition, Gillings School of Global Public Health, The University of North Carolina at Chapel Hill, Chapel Hill, North Carolina, USA

CAITLIN A. HILDEBRAND, MD, MPH
Center for Health Promotion and Disease Prevention, Department of Nutrition, Gillings School of Global Public Health, The University of North Carolina at Chapel Hill, Chapel Hill, North Carolina, USA

DANIELA JODORKOVSKY, MD
Division of Digestive and Liver Diseases, Columbia University Irving Medical Center, New York, New York, USA

THOMAS C. KEYSERLING, MD, MPH
Center for Health Promotion and Disease Prevention, Division of General Medicine and Clinical Epidemiology, Department of Medicine, School of Medicine, The University of North Carolina at Chapel Hill, Chapel Hill, North Carolina, USA

JUDITH KORNER, MD, PhD
Division of Endocrinology, Diabetes and Metabolism, Professor, Department of Medicine, Vagelos College of Physicians and Surgeons, Columbia University Irving Medical Center, New York, New York, USA

PENNY M. KRIS-ETHERTON, PhD, RD, FAHA, FNLA, FASN, CLS
Evan Pugh University Professor of Nutritional Sciences, Department of Nutritional Sciences, The Pennsylvania State University, Pennsylvania, USA

NICOLE KUERZI, BS, RD, CDN, CNSC
Department of Food and Nutrition, NewYork-Presbyterian Hospital, Columbia University Irving Medical Center, New York, New York, USA

WALTER L. LARIMORE, MD
UCHealth Occupational Medicine Clinic, Colorado Springs, Colorado, USA

JIM MANN, MD, PhD
Professor, Department of Medicine, University of Otago, Dunedin, New Zealand

ELIZABETH MIRACLE, MS, RD, CSO, CDN, CNSC
Department of Food and Nutrition, NewYork-Presbyterian Hospital, Columbia University Irving Medical Center, New York, New York, USA

DÓNAL O'MATHÚNA, BSc(Pharm), MA, PhD
Associate Professor, College of Nursing, Helene Fuld Health Trust National Institute for Evidence-based Practice in Nursing and Healthcare, The Ohio State University, Columbus, Ohio, USA

ALEXANDER PANDA, MD, PhD, MPH
Scientist II, Jean Mayer USDA Human Nutrition Research Center on Aging,
Tufts University, Boston, Massachusetts, USA

KRISTINA PETERSEN, PhD, APD, FAHA
Assistant Professor, Department of Nutritional Sciences, Texas Tech University, Texas,
USA

SYDNEY POMENTI, MD
Division of Digestive and Liver Diseases, Columbia University Irving Medical Center,
New York, New York, USA

TIRISSA J. REID, MD
Division of Endocrinology, Diabetes and Metabolism, Assistant Professor, Department of
Medicine, Vagelos College of Physicians and Surgeons, Columbia University Irving
Medical Center, New York, New York, USA

ANDREW REYNOLDS, PhD
Department of Medicine, University of Otago, Dunedin, New Zealand

CONNIE J. ROGERS, PhD, MPH
Professor and Department Head, Department of Nutritional Sciences, University of
Georgia, Athens, Georgia, USA

CARMEN D. SAMUEL-HODGE, RD, PhD
Center for Health Promotion and Disease Prevention, Department of Nutrition, Gillings
School of Global Public Health, The University of North Carolina at Chapel Hill, Chapel Hill,
North Carolina, USA

R. DREW SAYER, PhD
Assistant Professor, Department of Nutrition Sciences, The University of Alabama at
Birmingham, Birmingham, Alabama, USA

CHINARA TATE, PhD, RD
Director of Nutrition, Department of Psychiatry, Eating and Weight Disorders Program in
Excellence, Icahn School of Medicine at Mount Sinai, New York, New York, USA

MELISSA TOWNSEND, MS, RD, CDN
Department of Food and Nutrition, NewYork-Presbyterian Hospital, Columbia University
Irving Medical Center, New York, New York, USA

TED WILSON, PhD
Department of Biology, Winona State University, Winona, Minnesota, USA

Contents

Both scientific evidence and popular diet trends have sought to identify the ideal diet for weight loss with strategies focused on either restricting carbohydrates or fat. While there is a strong physiologic rationale for either carbohydrate restriction or fat restriction to achieve a calorie deficit needed for weight loss, evidence from randomized controlled trials suggest either type of diet is effective for weight loss. The level of adherence, rather than macronutrient content, is the driver of successful weight loss.

Two of the leading chronic diseases are cardiovascular disease (CVD) and cancer. A cornerstone of prevention for CVD and cancer is a healthy dietary pattern throughout the lifespan. Dietary patterns represent the totality of the diet and reflect habitual consumption of combinations and quantities of foods and nutrients that cumulatively affect health and disease. This article summarizes recent evidence on the relationship of diet quality as measured by adherence to healthy dietary patterns and CVD and cancer risk reduction. Optimal adherence to a healthy dietary pattern decreases CVD and cancer risk; even small changes in diet quality are beneficial.

With the growing burden of diet-related chronic disease impacting the public's health, nutrition counseling in a primary care setting is essential and can be accomplished through brief and creative approaches. This article reviews an example of a brief dietary assessment and counseling tool and counseling strategies focusing on dietary behavior changes that emphasize impact on health outcomes, ease of behavior change, and affordability. These, plus integrating office supports, are practical ways to start the conversation about improving diet quality with patients. Collaborative efforts in nutrition care, particularly through collaboration with registered dietitians, present a valuable opportunity to meet the nutrition care needs of patients. Additionally, this article reviews screening for eating disorders, food insecurity, and dietary supplement use.

to consume nutrient-dense foods. Many older adults do not maintain proper hydration, so adequate water intake should also be encouraged. Most older adults have multiple chronic diseases that may influence their dietary intake and nutritional needs. However, currently, our understanding of how individual chronic diseases and their associated treatments influence dietary requirements is limited.

This article serves as an overview for selecting appropriate nutrition education resources for patients, families, caregivers, and care providers. Registered Dietitians provide high-quality, evidence-based nutrition care and serve an integral role in multidisciplinary teams. However, all healthcare practitioners should be aware of the importance of providing meaningful nutrition education. Recommendations and considerations for health care practitioners providing individualized nutrition education or for providing disease and language-specific patient education materials are detailed. In addition, a brief review of insurance coverage for nutrition support services, as well as considerations to make when selecting a qualified nutrition provider for patient referrals is specified.

Erratum

In the article, "Can't Miss Infections: Endocarditis, Cellulitis, Erysipelas, Necrotizing Fasciitis, Cholecystitis", by Kim Tartaglia in a May 2022 issue of *Medical Clinics*, Figures 3-5 were assigned incorrect legends.

Figure 3 was incorrectly labeled on page 540 as "clubbing". This is a "Splinter hemorrhage".

Present correct figure 3 and label here

Figure 4 was incorrectly labeled on page 540 as "Janeway lesions, Osler nodes" and is a "Schamroth sign, indicative of clubbing of the digits".

Present correct figure 4 and label here

Lastly, Figure 5 was incorrectly labeled on page 541 "Petechiae" and are "Janeway lesions, Osler Nodes".

Present correct figure 5 and label here

medical.theclinics.com

Foreword
What We Can and Should Do

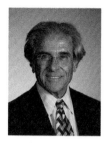

Jack Ende, MD, MACP
Consulting Editor

Mediterranean, ketogenic, or intermittent fasting? High fiber, low fiber, sodium restricted, or gluten-free? FODMAP restricted, vegan, low-carb, or DASH? These are just some of the publicized options promulgated for patients with assurance that a specific diet will lead to health, wellness, and even longevity.

Our patients, including those who are well and concerned most about maintaining their health, consume this information. Oftentimes they turn to us, their trusted health care providers, for guidance on what nutritional decisions are in their best interest.

Even more compelling are the questions we face in assisting our patients who have chronic illness. Diabetes, obesity, chronic kidney disease, hypertension, heart failure, and cancer, not to mention frailty, are just some of the important chronic illnesses that require astute nutritional management. How can and should we be advising these patients?

Our Guest Editor for this issue of *Medical Clinics of North America*, David Seres, offers in his accompanying Preface an astute appraisal of the state of knowledge in nutrition today. He is correct. The data do not always provide evidence-based answers for the questions our patients bring to us. But that is not to say the field of nutrition is bereft of sound guidance that we can and should be providing our patients. We can be reasonably certain of the important role nutrition plays in the aforementioned chronic illnesses. Even if all the answers are not available, we still should not ignore our patients' need for informed advice.

This, then, underscores the value of this remarkable issue of *Medical Clinics of North America*. Dr Seres and his authors provide insightful and comprehensive information and assemble for us the best evidence the field can provide. We all must admit that

Med Clin N Am 106 (2022) xvii–xviii
https://doi.org/10.1016/j.mcna.2022.08.008
0025-7125/22/© 2022 Published by Elsevier Inc.

medical.theclinics.com

nutrition has not always been at the forefront of medical practice. It is time for that to change.

Jack Ende, MD, MACP
Perelman School of Medicine of the
University of Pennsylvania
5033 West Gates Pavilion
3400 Spruce Street
Philadelphia, PA 19104, USA

E-mail address:
jack.ende@uphs.upenn.edu

Preface

Making Nutrition Accessible to the Generalist

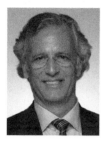

David S. Seres, MD, ScM, PNS, FASPEN
Editor

Dear Reader:

We hope that this issue will make nutrition accessible and understandable to the generalist. Nutrition is fascinating but can be frustrating. It is often confusing and counterintuitive. Generalists often report not knowing what to tell patients, and, if they believe they do, not knowing how to instruct them in such a way as to engender successful adherence. The quality of evidence is often very poor, given that most of what we believe comes from observational studies, so we nutrition experts often do not really know what to tell people, either.

It is easy to understand how nutrition is often felt to lack credibility when guidelines have changed so dramatically and frequently. I am often asked whether eggs are "in or out this time." While this usually engenders a smile when I mention it to trainees, the stakes could not be higher and the consequences more dire. People follow public health guidelines to live healthier and longer and disregard those who they feel have betrayed them.

From my perspective, as a nutrition support practitioner, finding high-quality evidence to drive the feeding of the sick or those with intestinal failure is no less daunting. Confusion abounds due to conflation of phenomena, such as the wasting of muscle due on the one hand to illness and on the other to starvation, into single syndromes. In this case, I refer to the term malnutrition, which is often not equivalent to being malnourished (see the Malnutrition and Enteral Nutrition article for a more robust discussion of this).

Fortunately, the iconoclastic view, that randomized control trials are the appropriate source for data to determine causal relationships, is gaining traction in nutrition.

In this issue, the authors and I have strived to provide a practical evidence-based guide for the generalist. I have gathered some of those most expert and experienced

Med Clin N Am 106 (2022) xix–xx
https://doi.org/10.1016/j.mcna.2022.07.011
0025-7125/22/© 2022 Published by Elsevier Inc.

in their field, but also authors willing to write transparently. We have endeavored to ensure the authors call out where the quality of evidence is high and low.

One very important article is missing. That being the article on sodium. Unfortunately, the author had health challenges that precluded completion in time for it to be included. So much has changed in the field. Now, huge cohort studies (mind you, they are still observational) suggest that our guidelines for sodium restriction may in fact be harmful. All of the world's heart associations, with the exception of the American Heart Association, have changed their recommendations from strict restriction (eg, 1500 mg) to avoiding excess (eg, <5000 mg). The new discovery of a large sodium storage system in the skin explains the lack of substantial blood pressure rise when sodium is loaded in normal volunteers and also explains why patients with heart failure go into pulmonary edema with a slice of pizza. Dietary sodium is rapidly scavenged and bound to glycosaminoglycans and becomes nonosmotic. In patients with hyperaldosteronemic states, such as those with heart failure, the storage system becomes saturated and dietary sodium remains oncotic.

It is our hope that this issue provides a practical tool and helps the reader better understand how to apply nutrition in any medical or surgical practice.

David S. Seres, MD, ScM, PNS, FASPEN
Columbia University Irving Medical Center
630 West 168th Street, P&S 9-501
New York, NY 10032, USA

E-mail address:
dseres@columbia.edu

The Data Behind Popular Diets for Weight Loss

Sarah E. Ehrlicher, PhD, RD[a,*], Tsz-Kiu Chui, MS, RD[b], Julianne G. Clina, MS[b], Katie M. Ellison, MS, RD[b], R. Drew Sayer, PhD[c]

KEYWORDS

- Weight loss • Low-carbohydrate diets • Low-fat diets • Diet adherence
- Appetite control • Cognitive restraint

KEY POINTS

- Both low-carbohydrate and low-fat diets (LFD) are effective for weight loss.
- Level of adherence to a calorie-restricted diet, rather than macronutrient content, is the driver of successful weight loss in the long term (>12 months).
- Strategies to control appetite and feelings of deprivation are important for improving adherence to a calorie-restricted diet for weight loss.

INTRODUCTION

The scientific community continues to put a considerable effort into understanding the effect of diet composition on the development, prevention, and treatment of obesity. All the while, the general population demands to know the secrets to weight loss. Numerous diet trends are popularized for weight loss despite the continued debate in the scientific community over the exact dietary causes of obesity. Both scientific and popular opinions on the ideal diet for weight loss and health have largely focused on the putative benefits and/or harms of dietary fat and carbohydrates, resulting in the "diet wars."

The landmark Framingham Heart study[1] in the 1950s and Seven Countries study[2] in the 1970s provided observational data linking saturated fat and cholesterol consumption to cardiovascular disease. These data led to recommendations by the American Heart Association and Academy of Nutrition and Dietetics for Americans to limit dietary fat intake. Soon after, the media publicized the "war on fat" with *Times* magazine publishing a cover story in 1984 about the dangers of cholesterol and the

---

[a] Department of Nutrition Sciences, University of Alabama at Birmingham, Webb 256, 1675 University Boulevard, Birmingham, AL 35294, USA; [b] Department of Nutrition Sciences, University of Alabama at Birmingham, Webb 630, 1675 University Blvd, Birmingham, AL 35294, USA; [c] Department of Nutrition Sciences, University of Alabama at Birmingham, Webb 634, 1675 University Boulevard, Birmingham, AL 35294, USA
* Corresponding author.
E-mail address: sehrlich@uab.edu

Med Clin N Am 106 (2022) 739–766
https://doi.org/10.1016/j.mcna.2022.05.003
0025-7125/22/© 2022 Elsevier Inc. All rights reserved.

recommendations to lower dietary fat intake.[3] As a result, dietary carbohydrate consumption in America increased by roughly 20% from 1970 to 1999.[4] However, despite the lower dietary fat intake, obesity rates continued to rise and may have even accelerated.[5] The implication to the scientific community was that the substitution of carbohydrates for fat in our food supply may have contributed to the obesity epidemic,[6] a notion supported by the association between increased consumption of sugar-sweetened beverages and weight gain.[7,8] Outspoken critics, such as Gary Taubes, blamed refined sugars in processed foods and sugar-sweetened beverages for the obesity epidemic, creating a "war on sugar."[9] In response, more popular diets arose with an emphasis on restricting carbohydrates and processed foods. Once again *Times* magazine exemplified this popular opinion with a cover story in 2014 on how scientists got it wrong by blaming fat for our health problems.[10]

In reality, both sides of the "diet wars" are likely misguided or at least incomplete descriptions of the role of diet composition in obesity development and treatment. It is much more likely that the highly palatable and energy-dense combination of fat and refined sugars promotes the overconsumption of calories, which—especially when coupled with decreases in energy expenditure—leads to weight gain and obesity.[11] There is now a growing consensus that there is no singular "ideal" diet for weight loss, and macronutrient distribution is only one factor in building a healthy dietary pattern.[12] Nonetheless, carbohydrate restriction has been an enduring trend in popular diets. Here we will discuss the physiologic rationale for considering macronutrient distribution for weight loss. Then, we will discuss a selection of several popular carbohydrate-restricted diets and the evidence that supports their use in weight loss. Additionally, we will discuss the comparison between low-fat and low-carbohydrate diets (LCD) for weight loss. Lastly, we provide a discussion of glycemic status as a possible predictor of weight loss and the biological and behavioral influencers on adherence as additional considerations for choosing a diet.

BACKGROUND: ENERGY BALANCE AND PHYSIOLOGIC RATIONALE FOR CARBOHYDRATE OR FAT RESTRICTION

In its simplest terms, the energy balance equation is made up of 3 components: energy intake, energy expenditure and energy storage.[13] When energy intake is greater than energy expenditure, the result is energy storage primarily as triglycerides in adipose tissue, which can eventually result in obesity.[14] It is well-established that changes in dietary intake have the strongest impact on energy balance, and much of the emphasis of weight-loss interventions is on a reduction in energy intake through a reduced-calorie diet.[15–17]

There are proponents of the carbohydrate-insulin model (CIM) which supports a reduction in carbohydrate, and those that support a reduction in dietary fat for weight loss. The CIM of obesity hypothesizes that diets high in carbohydrates lead to obesity due to the resulting increase in insulin concentration during the postprandial period(reviewed in[18,19]). Insulin is a potent regulator of metabolic actions in tissues throughout the body that impact both energy intake and energy storage (**Fig. 1**). Insulin action in the postprandial state suppresses the release and oxidation of fatty acids and increases fat storage (reviewed in[20]). Specifically, insulin inhibits fatty acid oxidation in muscle tissue[21] resulting in decreased whole-body fat oxidation after the ingestion of a carbohydrate-rich meal.[22] Dietary carbohydrates are preferentially metabolized and inhibit signals of fat oxidation,[23] contributing to the likelihood that the fat in the meal will be stored rather than metabolized.[24] Insulin suppresses the activity of hormone-sensitive lipase in adipose tissue to decrease the rate of lipolysis resulting in

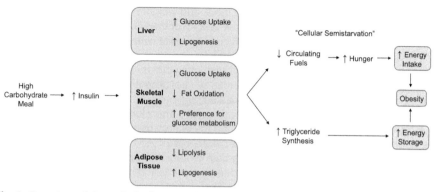

Fig. 1. Overview of the carbohydrate-insulin model (CIM) of obesity development. Ingestion of high carbohydrate meals causes large increases in circulating insulin, which has metabolic regulatory effects on various tissues throughout the body. In the liver, insulin increases glucose uptake and fatty acid synthesis (lipogenesis). In skeletal muscle, insulin increases glucose uptake and decreases fat oxidation leading to a preference for glucose metabolism. In adipose tissue, insulin decreases lipolysis and increases lipogenesis. Overall, insulin is promoting triglyceride synthesis from both dietary carbohydrates and fat and ultimately increased energy storage. The CIM posits that by the late postprandial period, the decrease in circulating fuels triggers a sense of "cellular semistarvation" that increases hunger and energy intake. The increases in energy intake and energy storage contribute to obesity.

decreased plasma free-fatty acid concentration.[25] Additionally, insulin increases lipogenesis and triglyceride synthesis in liver and adipose tissue from both dietary fat and carbohydrate because of the increased glucose and fatty acid uptake,[26] promoting energy storage. Consistent with this model is evidence that the initiation of exogenous insulin is associated with weight gain for those with type 1 or type 2 diabetes.[27,28] Insulin action to increase glucose and fatty acid uptake while simultaneously inhibiting the release of endogenous fatty acids and glucose leads to the decline in circulating metabolic fuels by the end of the postprandial period.[29] This decline in energy availability may be sensed by the central nervous system as a "cellular semistarvation" state that triggers an increase in hunger signals and energy intake.[19] In support of this theory, subjects reported higher hunger and consumed more calories during a meal test after hyperinsulinemic infusion in both hyperglycemic and hypoglycemic states, demonstrating that insulin is a driver of increased energy intake.[30] Altogether, insulin is responsible for altered substrate metabolism, resulting in the suppression of fat oxidation, promotion of energy storage and increased energy intake. Due to these physiologic effects of carbohydrates and insulin, the CIM posits that chronic ingestion of a high-carbohydrate diet may lead to excess adiposity and obesity.

Although there is a strong physiologic rationale for the detrimental effects of a high-carbohydrate diet inducing high insulin release, Hall and colleagues argue that the proposed CIM is not supported in clinical practice.[31] The CIM proposes that insulin suppresses fat metabolism to an extent that significantly impairs fat loss during weight loss, but results from multiple studies provide contradictory evidence. For example, highly controlled feeding studies have demonstrated that carbohydrate restriction did increase fat oxidation (as predicted by the CIM), but this did not lead to greater loss of fat mass compared with a low-fat/high-carbohydrate diet. In fact, fat loss was greater when participants consumed a low-fat diet (LFD) in both studies.[32,33] A 2-year weight loss clinical trial comparing LCD with LFD demonstrated that reductions in body weight and fat mass do not differ between diet types at any time points, with groups losing equivalent amounts of fat mass and weight regardless of carbohydrate intake.[34] These clinical studies testing the validity of the CIM support that weight loss is a complex physiologic state that is difficult to predict with a single factor though calorie restriction is the main driver of weight loss.

There is also a physiologic rationale for restricting dietary fat to minimize weight gain and lower the risk for obesity which includes several potential reasons. Fat is the most energy-dense macronutrient and provides 9 kcals per gram compared with carbohydrates and protein which provide 4 kcals per gram. Therefore, lowering the fat content of foods has the greatest effect on lowering the energy density of foods, which is recommended to help with adherence to a calorie-restricted diet.[35] Additionally, energy derived from dietary fat is less satiating than dietary carbohydrates, which promotes passive overconsumption and is argued to be a primary driver of positive energy balance and weight gain.[36,37] Studies have also demonstrated that while carbohydrate intake stimulates carbohydrate oxidation, ingesting fat does not immediately increase fat oxidation.[38,39]

Some slight differences between fat and carbohydrate digestion are also suggested reasons for limiting dietary fat. Fat is thought to be more readily absorbed and cause less of diet-induced thermogenesis compared with carbohydrates, so that greater net energy is extracted from dietary fat (reviewed in[40]). Although there is evidence to suggest these slight differences in macronutrient digestion may not be physiologically significant.[11] Altogether, there is a rationale that a LFD coupled with calorie restriction would successfully prevent and treat obesity.

CURRENT EVIDENCE: POPULAR CARBOHYDRATE-RESTRICTED DIETS VERSUS LOW-FAT DIETS FOR WEIGHT LOSS

Weight loss is effective for treating and preventing the progression of various cardio-metabolic diseases whereby weight loss of greater than 5% of initial body weight is considered clinically significant.[41] Carbohydrate restriction is a primary component for many popular diets aimed at weight loss. The Banting diet, described by William Banting in the 1800s, was the first LCD introduced for weight loss.[42] Banting chronicled his personal weight loss journey in a published pamphlet in which he followed a high-protein diet and eliminated foods high in starch and sugar and concluded that this diet would be the cure to obesity. Since then, numerous popular LCDs have been created that promote a similar message with slightly different diet compositions. **Table 1** provides descriptions for a selection of popular LCDs. Although a diet may become popular among the general public, not all popular LCDs have been rigorously studied to test their effectiveness for weight loss. An example of this is the Whole 30 diet which was popularized in the late 2000s as a quick crash diet to lose weight through the strict elimination of most carbohydrate foods including added sugar, grains, and legumes.[43] Whole 30 has not been studied in observational or randomized control trials for its effectiveness or benefits compared with any other weight loss diet. Among those that have been studied, few have strong evidence supporting the claims, while a majority have weak evidence that requires more ongoing research. An early meta-analysis investigating the effect of popular diets on weight loss observed an average of 8.73 kg weight loss after 6 months in LCDs, including the Atkins and Zone diets, though the weight loss did not significantly differ between tested popular diets.[44] A more recent meta-analysis observed a time effect, whereby modest weight reductions were seen at 6 months with the Atkins (5.5 kg) Zone (4.1 kg) and Paleo (5.3 kg) diets, but the effects diminished at 12 months due to weight regain.[45] Together, these analyses suggest popular LCDs are effective for weight loss in the

Table 1
Descriptions of select popular carbohydrate-restricted diets

Diet	Year	Brief Description	Diet Composition
Banting[42]	1863	First introduced by William Banting for weight loss. • Low carbohydrate, high fat, high protein • Avoid foods high in starch and sugar	Unspecified
Atkins Diet[46,47]	1970s	Developed by Dr Robert Atkins, M.D. Emphasis is low carbohydrate content of varying gram amounts depending on the level of restriction: • Atkins 20®: 20g net carbs/d • Atkins 40®: 40g net carbs/d • Atkins 100®: 100g net carbs/d Encourage foods high in protein and unsaturated fats but do not limit saturated fat intake.	25% protein 10% CHO 65% fat (Depends on levels of restriction)
Zone Diet[47,55]	1990s	Developed by Barry Sears, Ph.D. • Encourage fruits & vegetables, whole grains, lean protein, monounsaturated fat, omega-3 fatty acids • Eliminate foods that are high in sugar and starch including bread, pasta, grains • Eliminate saturated fat from red meat, egg, organ meats, and processed foods	30% protein 40% CHO 30% fat
Paleo Diet[47,59]	2000s	Mimic food groups from hunter-gatherer ancestors: • Features meat, nuts, eggs, healthy oil, fresh fruits, and vegetables • Eliminates processed/refined products such as cereal grains, legumes, and dairy • Low ratio of omega-6 to omega-3	30% protein 40% CHO 30% fat
South Beach diet[44,63]	2003	Developed by Dr Arthur Agatston, M.D. Phase 1 (2 wk): Weight loss • Restrict certain types of carbohydrates including bread, potatoes, pasta, baked goods, fruits, sweets, and so forth. Phase 2: Encourage lean protein and low-fat dairy, and gradually reintroduce certain carbohydrates and fruits Phase 3: Continue phase 2 and expand the quantity and selection of carbohydrates.	~30% protein ≤40% CHO 30%–55% fat
Whole30[43]	2009	Developed by Melissa Urban and Dallas Hartwig. Diet lasts for 30 d and eliminated food can be reintroduced after 30 d. • Eliminates added sugars, alcohol, grains, most legumes, dairy, and food additives	Unspecified

(continued on next page)

Table 1 (continued)			
Diet	Year	Brief Description	Diet Composition
Ketogenic Diet[47]	2010s	Very similar to Atkins diet. Initially introduced to treat patients with epilepsy in 1920s. Starting 2010s, gained popularity for weight loss.	20% protein 10% CHO ($\leq$50 g/d) 70% fat

Abbreviation: CHO, carbohydrate.

short-term with minimal differences between diets. In the following section, we will discuss current evidence on selected popular LCDs and **Table 2** provides descriptions and main findings of selected randomized clinical trials (RCT).

Atkins Diet

The Atkins diet is a very-LCD with versions prescribing as low as 20 g of net carbohydrates per day (see **Table 1** [46,47]). Current evidence suggests that the Atkins diet produces the greatest amount of weight loss by 6 months, but there is either minimal additional weight loss or likelihood of some weight regain between 6 months and 12 months (see **Table 2** [34,48–54]). Evidence for effects beyond 12 months is limited but the effectiveness seems to be mixed and heavily influenced by adherence. Shai, and colleagues, found that overall weight loss at 24 months remained significantly greater in the Atkins group compared with a LFD group (-4.7 ± 6.5 kg vs -2.9 ± 4.2 kg, $P<.001$) despite lower adherence rates (78% Atkins vs 90.4% LFD).[53] However, Foster and colleagues found that weight loss diminished between 12 and 24 months in the Atkins group and was not significantly different from the LFD group at 24 months (-6.34 kg vs -7.37 kg, $P = .41$).[34] Two other studies did not find significant differences in weight loss between Atkins and control diets at 12 months, which was attributed to decreased adherence to the Atkins diet over time.[50,54] When compared with other popular LCDs, meta-analyses suggest that the Atkins diet resulted in the greatest amount of weight loss at 6 months with one study estimating an effect of 10.12 kg[44] and another study estimating an effect of 5.46 kg.[45] However, the estimated effects decreased to 6.36 kg[44] and 3.84 kg[45] at 12 months.

Zone Diet

The Zone diet is a LCD with equal proportions of protein and fat (see **Table 1** [47,55]). Current evidence suggests that the Zone Diet is effective for producing significant weight loss in the short term (<12 months), but no studies have looked beyond 1 year (see **Table 2** [50,52,56,57]). The greatest observed weight loss from the Zone Diet was observed in 2 RCTs with -9.1 kg at 4 months[56] and -9.3 kg at 12 months,[57] although this effect was not significantly different from the high carbohydrate control diets. Meta-analyses suggest that the Zone Diet resulted in the estimated weight loss effect of 8.44 kg and 4.07 kg weight loss at 6 months.[44,45] Similar to the Atkins diet, the weight loss effects of the Zone Diet decreased to 5.95 kg and 3.25 kg at 12 months.[44,45]

Paleo Diet

The Paleo diet was designed to mimic the eating patterns of our early hunter-gatherer ancestors with high animal protein and complete elimination of refined grain products[58] (see **Table 1** [47,59]). Available evidence suggests that following the Paleo diet may be effective for weight loss (see **Table 2** [60,61]). For short-term effects, the Paleo diet showed significantly more weight loss at 1, 6, and 12 months when compared with a control diet.[60,61] For long-term effects, one RCT found that weight loss did not differ from the control diet at 24 months.[60] Meta-analyses of studies suggested that the Paleo diet resulted in greater overall weight loss of −3.52 kg (95% CI: -5.26 to −1.79, P<.001) compared with control diets.[62] Following the Paleo diet *ad libitum* resulted in a greater energy deficit compared with control diet (−20% vs −12%),[60] which is suggested to be mediated by the satiating effects of the high protein foods and low-energy-dense foods. However, the lack of weight loss difference at 24 months compared with control suggests that adherence to the diet decreased over time and the energy deficit was diminished.

South Beach Diet

The South Beach diet is a moderate carbohydrate diet that restricts mainly starchy and sweet foods and restricted foods can be later introduced back into the diet after 2 weeks (see **Table 1** [47,63]). Currently, evidence is limited to support the effect of the South Beach diet on weight loss (see **Table 2**). One RCT was conducted in patients after gastric bypass surgery and found that following the South Beach diet resulted in significant weight loss after 3, 6, and 12 months, but the effect was not different from the control diet.[64] A meta-analysis suggested that the South Beach diet has estimated effects of 9.86 kg weight loss at 6 months from this one RCT study.[44]

Ketogenic Diet

The Ketogenic diet is now one of the most popular carbohydrate-restricted diets. It was initially introduced to treat patients with epilepsy in the 1920s but gained popularity for weight loss due to its similarity to the Atkins diet (see **Table 1** [47]). Current evidence suggests that the ketogenic diet shows promising results for short-term weight loss (<12 months) among individuals who are overweight or obese and/or have type 2 diabetes (T2DM) (see **Table 2** [65–73]). RCT studies showed that the ketogenic diet produced significantly more weight loss at 6 months when compared with a control diet.[67,70] However, weight loss did not differ at 6, 12, and 24 months when energy intake was matched between the ketogenic diet and control diet.[65,66,69] A recent meta-analysis suggested that the ketogenic diet resulted in significantly greater weight loss (−7.78 kg in individuals with T2DM, P<.001; 3.81 kg in overall individuals, P = .01) when compared with control diet.[74] When compared with diets containing different levels of carbohydrate restriction, one study found that the ketogenic diet did not result in a greater amount of weight loss but had lower rates of adherence,[73] suggesting that a very low carbohydrate diet is more challenging to follow and not necessary for clinically significant weight loss.

Low-Fat Versus Low-Carbohydrate Diets

For decades, dietary patterns consisting of 20% to 35% kcals from fat have been the public health recommendation published in the Dietary Guidelines for Americans.[75] An LFD is generally agreed to be less than 30% kcals from fat. A meta-analysis of studies comparing LFD with controls found that the LFD prevents weight gain in people at a normal weight and produces weight loss in people with obesity.[76] This was substantiated by 2 other meta-analyses, with one finding that for every 1% decrease in energy from fat, there was a 0.28 kg decrease in body weight,[77] and another finding that a 10% reduction in fat energy was associated with a weight change of −16 gm/d. 78 Nonetheless, numerous other meta-analyses and systematic reviews (SR), have shown that a diet low in carbohydrates and higher in fat is more effective in producing weight loss compared with LFDs[79–87] (**Table 3**). These studies consistently found that

Table 2
Characteristics and main findings of randomized trials for select popular diets

Study	Diet	Duration (Months)	Population	N	BMI Mean (SD) Kg/m²	Weight Change
Atkins Diet						
Foster et al,[48] 2003	Atkins vs LFD	12	Obese, otherwise healthy	63	Atkins: 33.9(3.8) Control: 34.4(3.1)	Atkins vs LFD %BW mean ± SD 3 mo: −6.8 ± 5.8 vs −2.7 ± 3.7, $P = .001$ 6 mo: −7.0 ± 6.5 vs −3.2 ± 5.6, $P = .02$ 12 mo: −4.4 ± 6.7 vs −2.5 ± 6.3, $P = .26$
Brehm et al,[49] 2003	Atkins vs LFD	6	Obese female, otherwise healthy	53	Atkins: 33.2(1.83) Control: 34.0(1.83)	Atkins vs LFD mean ± SD kg 3 mo: −7.6 ± 0.7 vs −4.2 ± 0.8, $P<.001$ 6 mo: −8.5 ± 1.0 kg vs −3.9 ± 1.0, $P<.001$
Dansinger et al,[50] 2005	Atkins, Zone, Weight watchers (WW), Ornish (low-fat)	12	Overweight or obese with 1 metabolic or cardiac risk factor	160	Atkins: 35(3.5) Zone: 34(4.5) WW: 35(3.8) Ornish: 35(3.9)	2 mo: mean ± SD kg Atkins: −3.6 ± 3.3; Zone: −3.8 ± 3.6; WW: −3.5 ± 3.8; Ornish: −3.6 ± 3.4; $P = .89$ 6 mo: mean ± SD kg Atkins: −3.2 ± 4.9; Zone: −3.4 ± 5.7; WW: −3.5 ± 5.6; Ornish: −3.6 ± 6.7; $P = .76$ 12 mo: mean ± SD kg Atkins: −2.1 ± 4.8; Zone: −3.2 ± 6.0; WW: −3.0 ± 4.9; Ornish: −3.3 ± 7.3; $P = .40$

Study	Duration (mo)	Diets	Population	N	BMI	Results
Truby et al,[51] 2006	6	Atkins, Slim-Fast, WW, Rosemary Conley (RC, low-fat)	Overweight or obese, otherwise healthy	293	Atkins: 31.9(2.2) WW: 31.2(2.7) Slim-Fast: 32.2(3.0) RC: 31.6(2.6) Control: 31.5(2.9)	2 mo: mean ± SD kg Atkins: −5.2 ± 4.4; WW: −4.7 ± 3.2; Slim-Fast: −3.7 ± 3.5; RC: −4.0 ± 3.3; Controls −0.4 ± 1.8; All diets vs Controls $P<.001$ 6 mo: mean ± SD kg Atkins: −6.0 ± 6.4; WW: −6.6 ± 5.4; Slim-Fast: −4.8 ± 5.6; RC: −6.3 ± 6.1; Controls: 0.6 ± 2.2; All diets vs Controls $P<.001$
Gardner et al,[52] 2007	12	Atkins, Zone, Ornish (low fat), LEARN (Prudent)	Overweight or obese, otherwise healthy	311	Atkins: 32.0(4.0) Zone: 31.0(3.0) Ornish: 32.0(3.0) LEARN: 31.0(4.0)	2 and 6 mo: amount of weight loss was not specified, but Atkins was significantly different than all other diet ($P<.001$) 12 mo: mean kg (95% CI) Atkins: −4.7 (−6.3, −3.); Zone −1.6 (−2.8, −0.4); Ornish −2.2 (−3.6,−0.8); LEARN -2.6 (−3.8, −1.3); Atkins was significantly different from Zone ($P = .01$) at 12 mo No significant difference among Zone, LEARN, and Ornish at any time points

(continued on next page)

Table 2
(continued)

Study	Diet	Duration (Months)	Population	N	BMI Mean (SD) Kg/m^2	Weight Change
Shai et al,[53] 2008	Atkins, Mediterranean (Med), LFD	24	Overweight or obese, T2DM or CVD	322	Atkins: 30.8(3.5) Med: 31.2(4.1) Control: 30.6(3.2)	Atkins vs LFD, mean ± SD kg −4.7 ± 6.5 vs −2.9 ± 4.2, P<.001 Med vs LFD mean ± SD kg −4.4 ± 6.0 vs −2.9 ± 4.2, P<.001
Davis et al,[54] 2009	Atkins, LFD	12	Overweight or obese with T2DM	105	Atkins: 35.0(6.0) Control: 37.0(6.0)	Atkins vs LFD, mean ± SD kg 3 mo: −5.2 ± 2.8 vs −3.2 ± 3.7 6 mo: −4.8 ± 3.5 vs −4.4 ± 5.3 12 mo: −3.1 ± 4.8 vs −3.1 ± 5.8
Foster et al,[34] 2010	Atkins, LFD	24	Obese, otherwise healthy	307	Atkins: 36.1(3.59) Control: 36.1(3.46)	Atkins vs LFD, mean kg (95% CI) 3 mo: −9.49 (−10.2, −8.85) vs.- 8.37 (−9.04, −7.71), P = .019 6 mo: −12.18 (−13.2, −11.2) vs −11.34(-12.4, −10.3), P = .25 12 mo: −10.87 (−12.1, 9.67) vs −10.81 (−12.4, −9.28), P = .95 24 mo: −6.34 (−8.06, −4.63) vs −7.37 (−9.10, −5.63), P = .41

Zone Diet

Source	Diets	Duration (mo)	Population	N	Baseline weight, kg	Results
Dansinger et al,[50] 2005	Atkins, Zone, WW, Ornish	12	Overweight or obese with 1 metabolic/cardiac risk factor	160	Atkins: 35(3.5) Zone: 34(4.5) WW: 35(3.8) Ornish: 35(3.9)	2 mo: mean ± SD kg Atkins: −3.6 ± 3.3; Zone: −3.8 ± 3.6; WW: −3.5 ± 3.8; Ornish: −3.6 ± 3.4; $P = .89$ 6 mo: mean ± SD kg Atkins: −3.2 ± 4.9; Zone: −3.4 ± 5.7; WW: −3.5 ± 5.6; Ornish: −3.6 ± 6.7; $P = .76$ 12 mo: mean ± SD kg Atkins: −2.1 ± 4.8; Zone: −3.2 ± 6.0; WW: −3.0 ± 4.9; Ornish: −3.3 ± 7.3; $P = .40$
Gardner et al,[52] 2007	Atkins, Zone, Ornish (low fat), LEARN (Prudent)	12	Overweight or obese, otherwise healthy	311	Atkins: 32.0(4.0) Zone: 31.0(3.0) Ornish: 32.0(3.0) LEARN: 31.0(4.0)	2 and 6 mo: amount of weight loss was not specified, but Atkins was significantly different than all other diets ($P<.001$). 12 mo: mean kg (95% CI) Atkins: −4.7 (−6.3, −3.); Zone −1.6 (−2.8, −0.4); Ornish −2.2 (−3.6,−0.8); LEARN -2.6 (−3.8, −1.3). Atkins was significantly different from Zone ($P = .01$) at 12 mo. No significant difference among Zone, LEARN and Ornish at any time points.

(continued on next page)

Table 2
(continued)

Study	Diet	Duration (Months)	Population	N	BMI Mean (SD) Kg/m²	Weight Change
Lasker et al,[56] 2008	Zone, HCD	4	Overweight or obese, otherwise healthy	65	Zone: 33.8(1.1) Control: 33.4(0.7)	Zone vs HCD: mean ± SD kg 4 mo: −9.1 ± 0.9 vs −6.9 ± 0.8, $P = .07$
Layman et al,[57] 2009	Zone, HCD	12	Overweight or obese, otherwise healthy	130	Zone: 32.2(0.5) Control: 32.7(0.5)	Zone vs HCD: mean ± SD kg 4 mo: −8.2 ± 0.5 vs −7.0 ± 0.5, $P>.05$ 12 mo: −9.3 ± 1.0 vs −7.4 ± 0.6, $P = .10$
Paleo Diet						
Mellberg et al,[60] 2014	Paleo, HCD	24	Overweight or obese postmenopausal female, otherwise healthy	70	Paleo: 32.7(3.6) Control: 32.6(3.3)	Paleo vs HCD: mean kg 12 mo: −8.7 vs −4.4, $P<.01$ 6 and 18 mo: amount of weight loss was not specified, but Paleo resulted in significantly more weight loss than control. 24 mo: amount of weight loss was not specified, but no significant difference reported between diets.
Genoni et al,[61] 2016	Paleo, Balanced (control)	1	Overweight female, otherwise healthy	39	All sample: 27.0(4.0)	Paleo vs Control: mean kg (95% CI) 1 mo: −3.2 (−3.8, −2.6) vs −1.21 (−2.0, −0.5), $P<.01$

South Beach Diet

Study	Diet	Duration (mo)	Population	N	BMI	Results
Swenson et al,[64] 2007	South Beach, LFD	12	Obese, Postgastric bypass surgery	32	Preoperative BMI South Beach: 50.7(8.7) Control: 46.3(9.4)	South Beach vs LFD, mean ± SD %BW 3 mo: −33.3 ± 8.9 vs −33.5 ± 8.9, $P = .95$ 6 mo: −50.8 ± 12.5 vs −51.0 ± 12.9, $P = .97$ 12 mo: −59.6 ± 13.0 vs −60.3 ± 15.3, $P = .96$

Ketogenic Diet

Study	Diet	Duration (mo)	Population	N	BMI	Results
Yancy et al,[67] 2004	Ketogenic, LFD	6	Obese, hyperlipidemic	120	Ketogenic: 34.0(5.2) Control: 34.6(4.9)	Ketogenic vs LFD: mean kg (95% CI) 6 mo: −12.0 (−13.8, −10.2) vs −6.5(-8.4, −4.6), $P<.001$
Brinkworth et al,[69] 2009	Ketogenic, LFD	12	Abdominal obesity with 1 other metabolic syndrome	118	Completers Ketogenic: 33.6(4.0) Control: 33.3(3.9)	Ketogenic vs LFD: mean ± SD kg 12 mo completers: −14.5 ± 1.7 vs −11.5 ± 1.2, $P = .14$
Yancy et al,[68] 2010	Ketogenic, LFD + Orlistat	12	Overweight with one obesity-related disease or obese regardless of comorbidity	146	Ketogenic: 39.9(6.9) Low fat + Orlistat: 38,8(7.0)	Ketogenic vs LFD + Orlistat: mean kg (95% CI) 48 wk: −11.37 (−14.84, −7.89) vs −9.62 (−11.94, −7.29), $P = .41$
Saslow et al,[71] 2014, Saslow et al,[70] 2017	Ketogenic, MCD	12	Overweight or obese with T2DM or prediabetes	34	Ketogenic: 36.2(8.2) Control: 37.4(6.4)	Ketogenic vs MCD: 3 mo: −5.5 kg vs −2.6 kg, $P = .09$ 6 mo: −7.1 ± 4.5%BW vs 2.7 ± 5.4%BW, $P = .02$ 12 mo: −8.3 ± 5.8%BW vs −3.8 ± 6.0%BW, $P = .05$

(continued on next page)

Table 2
(continued)

Study	Diet	Duration (Months)	Population	N	BMI Mean (SD) Kg/m²	Weight Change
Tay et al,[65] 2014, Tay et al,[66] 2018	Ketogenic, LFD	24	Overweight or obese with T2DM	115	All sample: 34.4(4.2)	Ketogenic vs LFD: 6 mo: mean ± SD kg −12.0 ± 6.3 vs −11.5 ± 5.5, $P = .57$ 24 mo, mean kg (95%CI): −6.8 (−8.8, −4.7) vs −6.6 (−8.8, −4.5), $P = .26$
Goday et al,[72] 2016	VLCK Low-calorie diet	4	Obese with T2DM	89	VLCK: 33.3(1.5) Control: 32.9(1.6)	Ketogenic vs Low-calorie: (kg) Amount of weight change was not specified, but VLCK diet resulted in significantly more weight loss at 4 mo compared with control, $P<.001$.
Harvey et al,[73] 2019	VLCKD LCD MCD	3	Overweight, otherwise healthy	77	VLCKD: 25.5(2.8) LCD: 29.1(4.9) MCD: 26.4(3.2)	3 mo: mean kg(95%CI) VLCKD: −4.1(5.6, −2.7); LCD: −3.9(-6.2,-1.7); MCD: −3.0(-5.0, −0.9); $P = .63$

Abbreviations: %BW, percent body weight; BMI, body mass index; CVD, cardiovascular disease; HCD, high-carbohydrate diet; LCD, low-carbohydrate diet; LFD, low-fat diet; MCD, moderately low carbohydrate diet; SD, standard deviation; T2DM, type 2 diabetes mellitus; VLCKD, very low-carbohydrate ketogenic diet; VLCK, very low-carbohydrate ketogenic diet; WW, weight watchers.

LCDs produce greater weight loss in the short term (<12 months) compared with LFDs. Some studies found a statistically significant advantage of LCDs beyond 12 months,[81,83,85] although mean differences between LCD and LFDs were estimated to be within 1 kg which may not be clinically significant.

Interestingly, one meta-analysis found a >99% probability of greater weight loss with an LCD than an LFD[84] yet, another found that weight loss was greater on the LFD for those who weighed 10 kg more than the average at baseline (2.6 ± 0.8 kg, $P = .011$).[76] However, it should be noted that this study compared LFD to participants' usual diet or medium-fat diets that may not have been low in carbohydrate which could explain why the authors concluded in favor of the LFD. When Tobias and colleagues compared LFDs to various other diets, they concluded that there was a greater weight change with the LFD when compared with participants' usual diets (−5.41 kg [-7.29, −3.54], $P = .003$), but not when compared with higher fat diets (0.36 kg [-0.66, 1.37], $P = .49$). In line with the other studies discussed here, they also observed significantly greater weight loss from LCD when compared with LFD (1.15 kg [0.52, 1.79], $P<.001$).[85] Overall, these data suggest restricting dietary fat may produce weight loss, but weight loss is consistently greater if carbohydrates are restricted. Macronutrient distribution is an important consideration, however, not necessarily more important than overall energy restriction. In the presence of an energy deficit, weight loss will occur regardless of a diet's composition.[88]

DISCUSSION

We ended the previous section with the conclusion that clinically significant weight loss can be achieved on an energy-restricted diet of either a low-fat or low-carbohydrate composition. Identifying the most beneficial diet pattern for weight loss requires additional considerations of other dietary components and adherence. A primary factor determining the success of a weight loss diet is the level of adherence that can be achieved by the individual.[89,90] A hallmark study supporting this notion is one from Sacks and colleagues which measured changes in weight over 2 years between 4 diets that differed in macronutrient composition.[91] The principal finding was that participants achieved and maintained clinically meaningful weight loss similarly on all 4 diets, regardless of emphasizing one macronutrient over another. Though the macronutrient composition differed, intensive behavioral counseling was provided consistently across groups. Importantly, attendance at group sessions strongly predicted weight loss at 2 years (−0.2 kg for every session attended), suggesting that commitment and adherence are the driving factors behind successful weight loss.

It is a common thought that willpower is the most important factor needed to adhere to a diet and achieve weight loss. Motivation and willingness are certainly necessary for a person to adhere to a weight loss program. However, there are a number of biological and behavioral factors that influence adherence and that can be barriers to weight loss and weight loss maintenance (**Fig. 2**).[92] Biology is altered after weight loss due to shifts in energy balance. Weight loss increases appetite[93] and lowers energy expenditure,[94] influencing both sides of the energy balance equation. The physiologic mechanisms underlying these compensatory changes affecting energy balance are reviewed in-depth elsewhere.[95] Here we will discuss how appetite control and psychological factors may affect adherence to a weight loss diet.

Appetite Control Influences Adherence

Appetite and hunger signals are increased in the short-term when energy intake is restricted[96] and after a short-term (4 or 8 weeks) weight loss,[97] increasing the drive

Table 3
Summary of systematic review and meta-analyses comparing low-fat and low-carbohydrate diets

Reference/Study Design	Diet Protocol	# Studies/Inclusion Criteria	Mean Difference in Weight Loss (95% CI)	Adherence/Attrition
Astrup et al,[79] 2000 MA of control trials	Ad libitum LFD vs habitual diet or medium-fat ad libitum	16 Total/14 RCTs 2–12 mo duration, adult population	Favored LFD 3.2 kg (1.9, 4.5), P<.0001	Not reported
Nordmann et al,[80] 2006 MA of RCTs	LCD (≤60 gm/d) vs LFD (<30% kcals fat)	5 ≥ 6 mo, BMI ≥ 25 kg/m², ITT analysis	Favored LCD 6 mo: −3.3 kg (−5.3, −1.4), P = .02 12 mo: −1.0 kg (−3.5, 1.5), P = .15	6 mo: LCD 70% more likely to complete study vs LFD (odds ratio: 1.8). No difference after 12 mo.
Hession et al,[81] 2009 SR of RCTs	LCD/high protein vs LFD/ low calorie	13 ≥ 6 mo, adult population, BMI ≥ 28 kg/m²	Favored LCD 6 mo: −4.02 kg (−4.54, −3.49), P<.001 12 mo: −1.05 kg (−2.09, −0.01), P<.001	Attrition rate of 36% when combining all studies. Significant difference in attrition between the 2 diets, P = .001.
Hu et al,[82] 2012 MA of RCTs	LCD (<45% kcals CHO) vs LFD (<30% kcals fat)	23 ≥ 6 mo duration, adult population	No difference −1.0 kg (−2.2. 0.2), P>.05	Not reported
Bueno et al,[83] 2013 MA of RCTs	VLCKD (≤50 gm carb/d) vs LFD (<30% kcals fat)	13 ≥ 12 mo follow-up, adult population	Favored VLCKD −0.91 kg (−1.65, −0.17), P = .02	Low adherence overall. During the follow-up period of most studies, CHO intake was higher than the diet protocol.
Sackner-Bernstein et al,[84] 2015 MA of RCTs	LCD (≤120 gm/d) vs LFD (<30% kcals fat)	17 ≥ 8 wk follow-up, adult population, BMI ≥ 25 kg/ m², no comorbidities other than dyslipidemia	Favored LCD −2.0 kg (−3.1, −0.9), P = .001,	Completion rates: 74.4% LCD vs 74.6% LFD.
Tobias et al,[85] 2015 SR and MA of RCTs	LFD (<30% kcals fat) vs other diets	53 Total 18 compared LCD for	Favored LFD when <0 LCD:1.15 kg (0.52, 1.79),	Not reported

Study	Comparison	N / Population	Weight loss	Comments
		weight loss >1-y, adult population	$P<.001$ Higher-fat diet: 0.36 kg (−0.66, 1.37), $P = .49$ Usual diet: −5.41 kg (−7.29, −3.54), $P = .003$	
Mansoor et al,[86] 2016 MA of RCTS	LCD (Atkins or <20% kcals CHO) vs LFD	11 ≥ 6 mo, ≥ 20 subjects per group, healthy adults	Favored LCD −2.17 kg (−3.36, −0.99), $P<.001$	Adherence decreased over time but was better in studies that emphasized behavioral treatment. Large variations in reported CHO intake, indicating poor adherence.
Chawla et al,[87] 2020 SR and MA of RCTs	LCD (<40% kcals CHO) vs LFD (<30% kcals fat)	38 Adult population without comorbidities	Favored LCD Overall: −1.00 kg (−1.53, −0.46), $P<.05$ 1–3 mo: −0.93 kg (−1.88, 0.02), $P>.05$ 3–6 mo: −1.47 kg (−3.85, 0.92), $P>.05$ 6–12 mo: −1.30 kg (−2.02, −0.57), $P<.05$ >12 mo: 0.83 kg (−0.95, 2.60), $P>.05$	Not reported

Abbreviations: BMI, body mass index; CHO, carbohydrate; ITT, intention-to-treat; LCD, Low-carbohydrate diet; LFD, low-fat diet; MA, meta-analysis; RCT, randomized control trial; SR, systematic review; VLCKD, very-low-carbohydrate ketogenic diet.

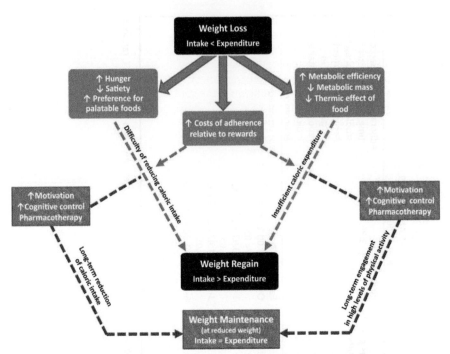

Fig. 2. Weight loss leads to both physiologic and psychological changes which promote subsequent weight regain (shown in *blue*). The path to overcome this propensity for regain (shown in *green*) may involve pharmaceutical and behavioral interventions that improve adherence, counter the physiologic and behavioral adaptations, and re-establish the balance between intake and expenditure. (*From* MacLean PS, Wing RR, Davidson T, et al. NIH working group report: Innovative research to improve maintenance of weight loss. Obesity (Silver Spring). Jan 2015;23(1):7-15. https://doi.org/10.1002/oby.20967 (*with permission*)[92].)

to eat on a calorie-restricted diet.[98] Therefore, adherence to a calorie-restricted diet is heavily influenced by the satiating effects of the diet and appetite control. It has been established that the macronutrient composition of meals influences satiety and appetite, whereby the dietary macronutrients have a hierarchical effect. When comparing carbohydrate-rich to fat-rich meals, ingestion of fat-rich meals has a weaker inhibitory effect on appetite and weaker promotion of satiety,[36,37,99] suggesting that high-fat/carbohydrate-restricted diets may increase the drive to eat and make it challenging to adhere to a calorie-restricted diet. However, in the case of very-low-carbohydrate and ketogenic diets, elevated ketone levels are considered a strong appetite suppressant[100] (reviewed in[101,102]). Carbohydrate-restricted diets may also be at a disadvantage if fiber content is low as high fiber content suppresses appetite and improves adherence.[103] A secondary analysis of the POUNDS Lost study found fiber content to be the most influential predictor of weight loss in participants consuming calorie-restricted diets of varying macronutrient compositions.[103] Additionally, a secondary analysis of the DIETFITS study made a direct comparison of fiber intake between LFD and LCD groups. Although the LFD group consumed significantly more fiber as expected, the difference was less than 4 g which are not expected to have a physiologically significant effect as weight loss was similar between groups,[104] suggesting that sufficient fiber content can be maintained on an LCD.

Protein has the strongest satiating effect compared with either carbohydrate or fat.[105–107] An LCD can be anywhere between 10% and 45% kcals from carbohydrate and this variability affects the relative contribution of protein. The weight loss effects of LCDs with increased protein content are thought to be primarily mediated by the satiating effects of the dietary protein and greater adherence to calorie restriction rather than the carbohydrate restriction per se.[108] One study used a 2 × 2 factorial design to investigate the effects of dietary protein and carbohydrate on weight loss.[109] Participants were assigned to one of the 4 groups for 12 months: low-carbohydrate/high-protein, low-carbohydrate/normal-protein, high-carbohydrate/high-protein, high-carbohydrate/normal-protein. At the end of the study, the high-protein groups had the greatest weight loss, suggesting that the differences in protein intake rather than carbohydrate intake were responsible for observed differences in weight loss.[109]

Psychological Factors Affecting Adherence

Psychological factors, including food cravings, disinhibition, and cognitive restraint, influence diet adherence. Food cravings are an "intense desire to eat a specific food" and are a common experience in eating behavior.[110] Restricted eating, commonly used in weight-loss diets, is associated with increased cravings for the restricted foods.[111,112] One study measured the frequency of experiencing and acting on food cravings after a weight loss program.[113] Although cravings for high energy-dense foods increased in frequency after the diet program, greater weight loss was associated with lower energy intake in response to those cravings,[113] demonstrating that subjects with successful weight loss experienced more food cravings but also greater restraint than subjects with less weight loss. Though a later study conducted by the same group found decreased cravings after weight loss,[114] so the research is not clear on how cravings are altered with weight loss and if this may differ based on the type of calorie-restricted diet.

Restricted eating is also associated with disinhibition (overeating when exposed to highly palatable foods or in response to emotional stress).[115] Cognitive restraint is the conscious effort needed to limit intake when presented with restricted foods.[111] It seems that those with greater weight loss in the short-term experience increased cognitive restraint, decreased disinhibition and decreased hunger.[116] However, in the long term, having higher cognitive restraint is associated with greater weight regain[117] because the high cognitive restraint is associated with loss of control and overeating when exposure to restricted foods inevitably occurs. Therefore, having lower feelings of deprivation is associated with greater weight loss.[118] Many of the popular diets for weight loss follow strict rules for complete elimination of certain foods and/or food groups (ie, dairy, grains, added sugar). Feelings of deprivation and restriction during a short-term weight loss diet have a psychological effect that is important to consider for the success of the weight loss diet and for the overall well-being of patients. Greater self-efficacy improves adherence and satisfaction with a restricted diet.[119] Strategies for improving self-efficacy is an area for potential individualization whereby a patient may feel less restricted and deprived, and therefore be more adherent, if they choose a calorie-restricted diet that matches their taste and cultural preferences. Further research is needed to understand how the restrictions of popular diets contribute to the psychological effects of adherence.

Glycemic Status as a Predictor of Weight Loss

Due to the variability in achieved weight loss that is typically observed in intervention trials, a new school of thought has emerged to consider how pretreatment biological status influences weight-loss success. Given the role that glucose and insulin play in energy regulation, numerous secondary analyses of weight-loss interventions have investigated whether pretreatment glycemia and insulinemia status can be used as predictors of weight loss. Evidence suggests that 3 distinct groups exist that respond differently given the same intervention: individuals with normoglycemia (fasting plasma glucose [FPG] <100 mg/dL), prediabetes (FPG 100–125 mg/dL), and T2DM (FPG ≥ 126 mg/dL). Hjorth and colleagues conducted retrospective analyses of three weight-loss interventions and found that those with normoglycemia tended to lose more or regain less weight on an LFD compared with LCD, whereas those with T2DM lost significantly more weight on an LCD compared with LFD.[120] Interestingly, an additional analysis demonstrated that people with prediabetes tend to respond differently depending on their fasting insulin (FI) values.[121] Those with low pretreatment FI but elevated FPG tended to lose more weight or maintain it longer on high fiber, moderate carbohydrate diets, whereas individuals with high pretreatment FI and FPG are more successful with an LCD. Those with normoglycemia but elevated FI tend not to respond differently by diet composition. Altogether, it seems that carbohydrate restriction may be beneficial for weight loss in people with high FPG and FI. These secondary analyses support using pretreatment biomarkers to predict individual responses to a low fat or LCD. The DIETFITS trial was designed to directly test this hypothesis. The DIETFITS trial assigned 609 adults aged 18 to 50 years with a BMI of 28 to 40 kg/m² to either an LFD or an LCD for 1 year.[122] On average, participants lost a similar amount of weight whether they were following an LFD or LCD and no significant diet-insulin secretion interaction effects were found. A separate SR attempted to test the effectiveness of LCDs for people with T2DM.[123] This analysis also concluded that it is likely no significant difference in changes in body weight between low-carbohydrate and balanced-carbohydrate diets in people with T2DM. Further research is needed on the use of pretreatment biomarkers to predict weight-loss response and to promote the use of diet in personalized medicine.

SUMMARY

While there is a strong physiologic rationale for either carbohydrate restriction or fat restriction to achieve a calorie deficit needed for weight loss, evidence from randomized control trials suggest that either type of diet is effective for weight loss. When directly comparing LFD to LCD, LCDs seem to be more effective in producing short-term weight loss, while differences in longer term weight loss may not be clinically significant. The popular Paleo and Ketogenic diets may produce a greater energy deficit when consumed *ad libitum* to promote weight loss in the short term, though adherence significantly decreases over time. Therefore, the level of adherence, rather than macronutrient content, is the driver of successful weight loss. Calorie-restricted diets for achieving weight loss can be individualized for patients to accommodate personal preferences in eating patterns and macronutrient composition to encourage greater long-term adherence.

CLINICS CARE POINTS

- Popular low-carbohydrate diets (LCD) are effective for weight loss and may offer greater short-term weight loss than low-fat diets (LFD).

- Low carbohydrate and LFD have similar weight-loss outcomes in the long term, suggesting no significant advantage of one over the other.
- Adherence to a calorie-restricted diet, rather than macronutrient composition, is a strong predictor of successful weight loss.
- Protein and fiber content are important for improving appetite control and adherence to a LCD.
- Psychological effects of restricted eating are important considerations for adherence and require more research to determine strategies for improving feelings of deprivation while on a calorie-restricted diet.
- Impaired glycemic status may be an indicator of better weight-loss outcomes from a LCD, though more research is needed to support this in clinical practice.

DISCLOSURE

The authors have nothing to disclose. Funding provided by General Mills (investigator-initiated grant), Nutrition Obesity Research Center grant P30 DK056336 and K01 DK124244.

REFERENCES

1. Dawber TR, Meadors GF, Moore FE Jr. Epidemiological approaches to heart disease: the Framingham Study. Am J Public Health Nations Health 1951;41(3):279–81.
2. Keys A, Blackburn H, Menotti A, et al. Coronary heart disease in seven countries. Circulation 1970;41:1–211.
3. Wallis C. Hold the eggs and butter. New York City, NY: Time; 1984. p. 56–63.
4. Carden TJ, Carr TP. Food availability of glucose and fat, but not fructose, increased in the U.S. between 1970 and 2009: analysis of the USDA food availability data system. Nutr J 2013;12:130.
5. Walker TB, Parker MJ. Lessons from the war on dietary fat. J Am Coll Nutr 2014;33(4):347–51.
6. Johnson RJ, Sanchez-Lozada LG, Andrews P, et al. Perspective: A Historical and Scientific Perspective of Sugar and Its Relation with Obesity and Diabetes. Adv Nutr 2017;8(3):412–22.
7. Malik VS, Schulze MB, Hu FB. Intake of sugar-sweetened beverages and weight gain: a systematic review. Am J Clin Nutr 2006;84(2):274–88.
8. Bray GA, Nielsen SJ, Popkin BM. Consumption of high-fructose corn syrup in beverages may play a role in the epidemic of obesity. Am J Clin Nutr 2004;79(4):537–43.
9. Taubes G. Good calories, bad calories. New York City, NY: Knopf Publishing; 2007.
10. Walsh B. Don't blame fat. New York City, NY: Time; 2014. p. 30–8.
11. Hall KD, Guo J. Obesity Energetics: Body Weight Regulation and the Effects of Diet Composition. Gastroenterology 2017;152(7):1718–1727 e3.
12. Pagoto SL, Appelhans BM. A call for an end to the diet debates. JAMA 2013;310(7):687–8.
13. Hill JO, Wyatt HR, Reed GW, et al. Obesity and the environment: where do we go from here? Science 2003;299(5608):853–5.
14. Hill JO, Wyatt HR, Peters JC. Energy balance and obesity. Circulation 2012;126(1):126–32.

15. Wadden TA. Treatment of obesity by moderate and severe caloric restriction. Results of clinical research trials. Ann Intern Med 1993;119(7 Pt 2):688–93.

16. Heilbronn LK, de Jonge L, Frisard MI, et al. Effect of 6-month calorie restriction on biomarkers of longevity, metabolic adaptation, and oxidative stress in overweight individuals: a randomized controlled trial. JAMA 2006;295(13):1539–48.

17. Curioni CC, Lourenco PM. Long-term weight loss after diet and exercise: a systematic review. Int J Obes (Lond) 2005;29(10):1168–74.

18. Ludwig DS, Ebbeling CB. The Carbohydrate-Insulin Model of Obesity: Beyond "Calories In, Calories Out. JAMA Intern Med 2018;178(8):1098–103.

19. Ludwig DS, Aronne LJ, Astrup A, et al. The carbohydrate-insulin model: a physiological perspective on the obesity pandemic. Am J Clin Nutr 2021. https://doi.org/10.1093/ajcn/nqab270.

20. Dimitriadis G, Mitrou P, Lambadiari V, et al. Insulin effects in muscle and adipose tissue. Diabetes Res Clin Pract 2011;93(Suppl 1):S52–9.

21. Kelley DE, Reilly JP, Veneman T, et al. Effects of insulin on skeletal muscle glucose storage, oxidation, and glycolysis in humans. Am J Physiol 1990;258(6 Pt 1):E923–9.

22. Surina DM, Langhans W, Pauli R, et al. Meal composition affects postprandial fatty acid oxidation. Am J Physiol 1993;264(6 Pt 2):R1065–70.

23. Kelley D, Mitrakou A, Marsh H, et al. Skeletal muscle glycolysis, oxidation, and storage of an oral glucose load. J Clin Invest 1988;81(5):1563–71.

24. Roberts R, Bickerton AS, Fielding BA, et al. Reduced oxidation of dietary fat after a short term high-carbohydrate diet. Am J Clin Nutr 2008;87(4):824–31.

25. Frayn KN, Shadid S, Hamlani R, et al. Regulation of fatty acid movement in human adipose tissue in the postabsorptive-to-postprandial transition. Am J Physiol 1994;266(3 Pt 1):E308–17.

26. Czech MP, Tencerova M, Pedersen DJ, et al. Insulin signalling mechanisms for triacylglycerol storage. Diabetologia 2013;56(5):949–64.

27. Carver C. Insulin treatment and the problem of weight gain in type 2 diabetes. Diabetes Educ 2006;32(6):910–7.

28. Carlson MG, Campbell PJ. Intensive insulin therapy and weight gain in IDDM. Diabetes 1993;42(12):1700–7.

29. Shimy KJ, Feldman HA, Klein GL, et al. Effects of Dietary Carbohydrate Content on Circulating Metabolic Fuel Availability in the Postprandial State. J Endocr Soc 2020;4(7):bvaa062.

30. Rodin J, Wack J, Ferrannini E, et al. Effect of insulin and glucose on feeding behavior. Metabolism 1985;34(9):826–31.

31. Hall KD, Guyenet SJ, Leibel RL. The Carbohydrate-Insulin Model of Obesity Is Difficult to Reconcile With Current Evidence. JAMA Intern Med 2018;178(8):1103–5.

32. Hall KD, Bemis T, Brychta R, et al. Calorie for Calorie, Dietary Fat Restriction Results in More Body Fat Loss than Carbohydrate Restriction in People with Obesity. Cell Metab 2015;22(3):427–36.

33. Hall KD, Chen KY, Guo J, et al. Energy expenditure and body composition changes after an isocaloric ketogenic diet in overweight and obese men. Am J Clin Nutr 2016;104(2):324–33.

34. Foster GD, Wyatt HR, Hill JO, et al. Weight and metabolic outcomes after 2 years on a low-carbohydrate versus low-fat diet: a randomized trial. Ann Intern Med 2010;153(3):147–57.

35. Rolls BJ. Dietary energy density: Applying behavioural science to weight management. Nutr Bull 2017;42(3):246–53.

36. Blundell JE, Burley VJ, Cotton JR, et al. Dietary fat and the control of energy intake: evaluating the effects of fat on meal size and postmeal satiety. Am J Clin Nutr 1993;57(5 Suppl):772S–7S [discussion: 777S-778S].

37. Cotton JR, Burley VJ, Weststrate JA, et al. Dietary fat and appetite: similarities and differences in the satiating effect of meals supplemented with either fat or carbohydrate. J Hum Nutr Diet 2007;20(3):186–99.

38. Flatt JP, Ravussin E, Acheson KJ, et al. Effects of dietary fat on postprandial substrate oxidation and on carbohydrate and fat balances. J Clin Invest 1985; 76(3):1019–24.

39. Schutz Y, Flatt JP, Jequier E. Failure of dietary fat intake to promote fat oxidation: a factor favoring the development of obesity. Am J Clin Nutr 1989;50(2):307–14.

40. Astrup A. The role of dietary fat in the prevention and treatment of obesity. Efficacy and safety of low-fat diets. Int J Obes Relat Metab Disord 2001;25(Suppl 1):S46–50.

41. Timothy Garvey W. New Horizons. A New Paradigm for Treating to Target with Second-Generation Obesity Medications. J Clin Endocrinol Metab 2022; 107(4):e1339–47.

42. Banting W. Letter on corpulence, addressed to the public. 1869. Obes Res 1993;1(2):153–63.

43. The Whole30 Program: Plan for Whole30 Success. Available at: https://whole30.com/whole30-program-rules/. Accessed March 30, 2022.

44. Johnston BC, Kanters S, Bandayrel K, et al. Comparison of weight loss among named diet programs in overweight and obese adults: a meta-analysis. JAMA 2014;312(9):923–33.

45. Ge L, Sadeghirad B, Ball GDC, et al. Comparison of dietary macronutrient patterns of 14 popular named dietary programmes for weight and cardiovascular risk factor reduction in adults: systematic review and network meta-analysis of randomised trials. BMJ 2020;369:m696.

46. Atkins Diet Mar 30, 2022. Available at: https://www.atkins.com/how-it-works/compare-plans. Accessed Mar 30, 2022.

47. Freire R. Scientific evidence of diets for weight loss: Different macronutrient composition, intermittent fasting, and popular diets. Nutrition 2020;69:110549.

48. Foster GD, Wyatt HR, Hill JO, et al. A randomized trial of a low-carbohydrate diet for obesity. N Engl J Med 2003;348(21):2082–90.

49. Brehm BJ, Seeley RJ, Daniels SR, et al. A randomized trial comparing a very low carbohydrate diet and a calorie-restricted low fat diet on body weight and cardiovascular risk factors in healthy women. J Clin Endocrinol Metab 2003;88(4): 1617–23.

50. Dansinger ML, Gleason JA, Griffith JL, et al. Comparison of the Atkins, Ornish, Weight Watchers, and Zone diets for weight loss and heart disease risk reduction: a randomized trial. JAMA 2005;293(1):43–53.

51. Truby H, Baic S, deLooy A, et al. Randomised controlled trial of four commercial weight loss programmes in the UK: initial findings from the BBC "diet trials. BMJ 2006;332(7553):1309–14.

52. Gardner CD, Kiazand A, Alhassan S, et al. Comparison of the Atkins, Zone, Ornish, and LEARN diets for change in weight and related risk factors among overweight premenopausal women: the A TO Z Weight Loss Study: a randomized trial. JAMA 2007;297(9):969–77.

53. Shai I, Schwarzfuchs D, Henkin Y, et al. Weight loss with a low-carbohydrate, Mediterranean, or low-fat diet. N Engl J Med 2008;359(3):229–41.

54. Davis NJ, Tomuta N, Schechter C, et al. Comparative study of the effects of a 1-year dietary intervention of a low-carbohydrate diet versus a low-fat diet on weight and glycemic control in type 2 diabetes. Diabetes Care 2009;32(7):1147–52.

55. The Zone Diet. Mar 30, 2022. Available at: https://zonediet.com/the-zone-diet/. Accessed March 30, 2022.

56. Lasker DA, Evans EM, Layman DK. Moderate carbohydrate, moderate protein weight loss diet reduces cardiovascular disease risk compared to high carbohydrate, low protein diet in obese adults: A randomized clinical trial. Nutr Metab (Lond) 2008;5:30.

57. Layman DK, Evans EM, Erickson D, et al. A moderate-protein diet produces sustained weight loss and long-term changes in body composition and blood lipids in obese adults. J Nutr 2009;139(3):514–21.

58. Konner M, Eaton SB. Paleolithic nutrition: twenty-five years later. Nutr Clin Pract 2010;25(6):594–602.

59. Cordain L, Eaton SB, Sebastian A, et al. Origins and evolution of the Western diet: health implications for the 21st century. Am J Clin Nutr 2005;81(2):341–54.

60. Mellberg C, Sandberg S, Ryberg M, et al. Long-term effects of a Palaeolithic-type diet in obese postmenopausal women: a 2-year randomized trial. Eur J Clin Nutr 2014;68(3):350–7.

61. Genoni A, Lyons-Wall P, Lo J, et al. Cardiovascular, Metabolic Effects and Dietary Composition of Ad-Libitum Paleolithic vs. Australian Guide to Healthy Eating Diets: A 4-Week Randomised Trial. Nutrients 2016;8(5).

62. de Menezes EVA, Sampaio HAC, Carioca AAF, et al. Influence of Paleolithic diet on anthropometric markers in chronic diseases: systematic review and meta-analysis. Nutr J 2019;18(1):41.

63. Agatston A. the South Beach diet: the delicious, doctor-designed, foolproof plan for fast and healthy weight loss. New York City, NY: St. Martin's Press; 2005.

64. Swenson BR, Saalwachter Schulman A, Edwards MJ, et al. The effect of a low-carbohydrate, high-protein diet on post laparoscopic gastric bypass weight loss: a prospective randomized trial. J Surg Res 2007;142(2):308–13.

65. Tay J, Luscombe-Marsh ND, Thompson CH, et al. A very low-carbohydrate, low-saturated fat diet for type 2 diabetes management: a randomized trial. Diabetes Care 2014;37(11):2909–18.

66. Tay J, Thompson CH, Luscombe-Marsh ND, et al. Effects of an energy-restricted low-carbohydrate, high unsaturated fat/low saturated fat diet versus a high-carbohydrate, low-fat diet in type 2 diabetes: A 2-year randomized clinical trial. Diabetes Obes Metab 2018;20(4):858–71.

67. Yancy WS Jr, Olsen MK, Guyton JR, et al. A low-carbohydrate, ketogenic diet versus a low-fat diet to treat obesity and hyperlipidemia: a randomized, controlled trial. Ann Intern Med 2004;140(10):769–77.

68. Yancy WS Jr, Westman EC, McDuffie JR, et al. A randomized trial of a low-carbohydrate diet vs orlistat plus a low-fat diet for weight loss. Arch Intern Med 2010;170(2):136–45.

69. Brinkworth GD, Noakes M, Buckley JD, et al. Long-term effects of a very-low-carbohydrate weight loss diet compared with an isocaloric low-fat diet after 12 mo. Am J Clin Nutr 2009;90(1):23–32.

70. Saslow LR, Daubenmier JJ, Moskowitz JT, et al. Twelve-month outcomes of a randomized trial of a moderate-carbohydrate versus very low-carbohydrate diet in overweight adults with type 2 diabetes mellitus or prediabetes. Nutr Diabetes 2017;7(12):304.

71. Saslow LR, Kim S, Daubenmier JJ, et al. A randomized pilot trial of a moderate carbohydrate diet compared to a very low carbohydrate diet in overweight or obese individuals with type 2 diabetes mellitus or prediabetes. PLoS One 2014;9(4):e91027.
72. Goday A, Bellido D, Sajoux I, et al. Short-term safety, tolerability and efficacy of a very low-calorie-ketogenic diet interventional weight loss program versus hypocaloric diet in patients with type 2 diabetes mellitus. Nutr Diabetes 2016;6(9): e230.
73. Harvey C, Schofield GM, Zinn C, et al. Low-carbohydrate diets differing in carbohydrate restriction improve cardiometabolic and anthropometric markers in healthy adults: A randomised clinical trial. PeerJ 2019;7:e6273.
74. Choi YJ, Jeon SM, Shin S. Impact of a Ketogenic Diet on Metabolic Parameters in Patients with Obesity or Overweight and with or without Type 2 Diabetes: A Meta-Analysis of Randomized Controlled Trials. Nutrients 2020;12(7). https://doi.org/10.3390/nu12072005.
75. U.S. Department of Agriculture and U.S. Department of Health and Human Services. Dietary Guidelines for Americans , 2020-2025. 9th edition. December 2020. Available at DietaryGuidelines.gov.
76. Astrup A, Grunwald GK, Melanson EL, et al. The role of low-fat diets in body weight control: a meta-analysis of ad libitum dietary intervention studies. Int J Obes Relat Metab Disord 2000;24(12):1545–52.
77. Yu-Poth S, Zhao G, Etherton T, et al. Effects of the National Cholesterol Education Program's Step I and Step II dietary intervention programs on cardiovascular disease risk factors: a meta-analysis. Am J Clin Nutr 1999;69(4):632–46.
78. Bray GA, Popkin BM. Dietary fat intake does affect obesity. Am J Clin Nutr 1998; 68(6):1157–73.
79. Astrup A, Ryan L, Grunwald GK, et al. The role of dietary fat in body fatness: evidence from a preliminary meta-analysis of ad libitum low-fat dietary intervention studies. Br J Nutr 2000;83(Suppl 1):S25–32.
80. Nordmann AJ, Nordmann A, Briel M, et al. Effects of low-carbohydrate vs low-fat diets on weight loss and cardiovascular risk factors: a meta-analysis of randomized controlled trials. Arch Intern Med 2006;166(3):285–93.
81. Hession M, Rolland C, Kulkarni U, et al. Systematic review of randomized controlled trials of low-carbohydrate vs. low-fat/low-calorie diets in the management of obesity and its comorbidities. Obes Rev 2009;10(1):36–50.
82. Hu T, Mills KT, Yao L, et al. Effects of low-carbohydrate diets versus low-fat diets on metabolic risk factors: a meta-analysis of randomized controlled clinical trials. Am J Epidemiol 2012;176(Suppl 7):S44–54.
83. Bueno NB, de Melo IS, de Oliveira SL, et al. Very-low-carbohydrate ketogenic diet v. low-fat diet for long-term weight loss: a meta-analysis of randomised controlled trials. Br J Nutr 2013;110(7):1178–87.
84. Sackner-Bernstein J, Kanter D, Kaul S. Dietary Intervention for Overweight and Obese Adults: Comparison of Low-Carbohydrate and Low-Fat Diets. A Meta-Analysis. PLoS One 2015;10(10):e0139817.
85. Tobias DK, Chen M, Manson JE, et al. Effect of low-fat diet interventions versus other diet interventions on long-term weight change in adults: a systematic review and meta-analysis. Lancet Diabetes Endocrinol 2015;3(12):968–79.
86. Mansoor N, Vinknes KJ, Veierod MB, et al. Effects of low-carbohydrate diets v. low-fat diets on body weight and cardiovascular risk factors: a meta-analysis of randomised controlled trials. Br J Nutr 2016;115(3):466–79.

87. Chawla S, Tessarolo Silva F, Amaral Medeiros S, et al. The Effect of Low-Fat and Low-Carbohydrate Diets on Weight Loss and Lipid Levels: A Systematic Review and Meta-Analysis. Nutrients 2020;12(12). https://doi.org/10.3390/nu12123774.

88. Stanhope KL, Goran MI, Bosy-Westphal A, et al. Pathways and mechanisms linking dietary components to cardiometabolic disease: thinking beyond calories. Obes Rev 2018;19(9):1205-35.

89. Del Corral P, Chandler-Laney PC, Casazza K, et al. Effect of dietary adherence with or without exercise on weight loss: a mechanistic approach to a global problem. J Clin Endocrinol Metab 2009;94(5):1602-7.

90. Alhassan S, Kim S, Bersamin A, et al. Dietary adherence and weight loss success among overweight women: results from the A TO Z weight loss study. Int J Obes (Lond) 2008;32(6):985-91.

91. Sacks FM, Bray GA, Carey VJ, et al. Comparison of weight-loss diets with different compositions of fat, protein, and carbohydrates. N Engl J Med 2009; 360(9):859-73.

92. MacLean PS, Wing RR, Davidson T, et al. NIH working group report: Innovative research to improve maintenance of weight loss. Obesity (Silver Spring) 2015; 23(1):7-15.

93. Sumithran P, Prendergast LA, Delbridge E, et al. Long-term persistence of hormonal adaptations to weight loss. N Engl J Med 2011;365(17):1597-604.

94. Redman LM, Heilbronn LK, Martin CK, et al. Metabolic and behavioral compensations in response to caloric restriction: implications for the maintenance of weight loss. PLoS One 2009;4(2):e4377.

95. Maclean PS, Bergouignan A, Cornier MA, et al. Biology's response to dieting: the impetus for weight regain. Am J Physiol Regul Integr Comp Physiol 2011; 301(3):R581-600.

96. Pasiakos SM, Caruso CM, Kellogg MD, et al. Appetite and endocrine regulators of energy balance after 2 days of energy restriction: insulin, leptin, ghrelin, and DHEA-S. Obesity (Silver Spring) 2011;19(6):1124-30.

97. Coutinho SR, With E, Rehfeld JF, et al. The impact of rate of weight loss on body composition and compensatory mechanisms during weight reduction: A randomized control trial. Clin Nutr 2018;37(4):1154-62.

98. Hintze LJ, Goldfield G, Seguin R, et al. The rate of weight loss does not affect resting energy expenditure and appetite sensations differently in women living with overweight and obesity. Physiol Behav 2019;199:314-21.

99. Hopkins M, Gibbons C, Caudwell P, et al. Differing effects of high-fat or high-carbohydrate meals on food hedonics in overweight and obese individuals. Br J Nutr 2016;115(10):1875-84.

100. Johnstone AM, Horgan GW, Murison SD, et al. Effects of a high-protein ketogenic diet on hunger, appetite, and weight loss in obese men feeding ad libitum. Am J Clin Nutr 2008;87(1):44-55.

101. Gibson AA, Seimon RV, Lee CM, et al. Do ketogenic diets really suppress appetite? A systematic review and meta-analysis. Obes Rev 2015;16(1):64-76.

102. Roekenes J, Martins C. Ketogenic diets and appetite regulation. Curr Opin Clin Nutr Metab Care 2021;24(4):359-63.

103. Miketinas DC, Bray GA, Beyl RA, et al. Fiber Intake Predicts Weight Loss and Dietary Adherence in Adults Consuming Calorie-Restricted Diets: The POUNDS Lost (Preventing Overweight Using Novel Dietary Strategies) Study. J Nutr 2019; 149(10):1742-8.

104. Offringa LC, Hartle JC, Rigdon J, et al. Changes in Quantity and Sources of Dietary Fiber from Adopting Healthy Low-Fat vs. Healthy Low-Carb Weight Loss

Diets: Secondary Analysis of DIETFITS Weight Loss Diet Study. Nutrients 2021; 13(10). https://doi.org/10.3390/nu13103625.

105. Halton TL, Hu FB. The effects of high protein diets on thermogenesis, satiety and weight loss: a critical review. J Am Coll Nutr 2004;23(5):373–85.

106. Westerterp-Plantenga MS, Lemmens SG, Westerterp KR. Dietary protein - its role in satiety, energetics, weight loss and health. Br J Nutr 2012;108(Suppl 2):S105–12.

107. Drummen M, Tischmann L, Gatta-Cherifi B, et al. Dietary Protein and Energy Balance in Relation to Obesity and Co-morbidities. Front Endocrinol (Lausanne) 2018;9:443.

108. Weigle DS, Breen PA, Matthys CC, et al. A high-protein diet induces sustained reductions in appetite, ad libitum caloric intake, and body weight despite compensatory changes in diurnal plasma leptin and ghrelin concentrations. Am J Clin Nutr 2005;82(1):41–8.

109. Soenen S, Bonomi AG, Lemmens SG, et al. Relatively high-protein or 'low-carb' energy-restricted diets for body weight loss and body weight maintenance? Physiol Behav 2012;107(3):374–80.

110. White MA, Whisenhunt BL, Williamson DA, et al. Development and validation of the food-craving inventory. Obes Res 2002;10(2):107–14.

111. Coelho JS, Polivy J, Herman CP. Selective carbohydrate or protein restriction: effects on subsequent food intake and cravings. Appetite 2006;47(3):352–60.

112. Hill AJ. The psychology of food craving. Proc Nutr Soc 2007;66(2):277–85.

113. Gilhooly CH, Das SK, Golden JK, et al. Food cravings and energy regulation: the characteristics of craved foods and their relationship with eating behaviors and weight change during 6 months of dietary energy restriction. Int J Obes (Lond) 2007;31(12):1849–58.

114. Batra P, Das SK, Salinardi T, et al. Relationship of cravings with weight loss and hunger. Results from a 6 month worksite weight loss intervention. Appetite 2013; 69:1–7.

115. Savage JS, Hoffman L, Birch LL. Dieting, restraint, and disinhibition predict women's weight change over 6 y. Am J Clin Nutr 2009;90(1):33–40.

116. Batra P, Das SK, Salinardi T, et al. Eating behaviors as predictors of weight loss in a 6 month weight loss intervention. Obesity (Silver Spring) 2013;21(11): 2256–63.

117. Liu X, Hanseman DJ, Champagne CM, et al. Predicting Weight Loss Using Psychological and Behavioral Factors: The POUNDS LOST Trial. J Clin Endocrinol Metab 2020;105(4). https://doi.org/10.1210/clinem/dgz236.

118. Sayer RD, Peters JC, Pan Z, et al. Hunger, Food Cravings, and Diet Satisfaction are Related to Changes in Body Weight During a 6-Month Behavioral Weight Loss Intervention: The Beef WISE Study. Nutrients 2018;10(6). https://doi.org/10.3390/nu10060700.

119. Cruwys T, Norwood R, Chachay VS, et al. "An Important Part of Who I am": The Predictors of Dietary Adherence among Weight-Loss, Vegetarian, Vegan, Paleo, and Gluten-Free Dietary Groups. Nutrients 2020;12(4). https://doi.org/10.3390/nu12040970.

120. Hjorth MF, Ritz C, Blaak EE, et al. Pretreatment fasting plasma glucose and insulin modify dietary weight loss success: results from 3 randomized clinical trials. Am J Clin Nutr 2017;106(2):499–505.

121. Hjorth MF, Bray GA, Zohar Y, et al. Pretreatment Fasting Glucose and Insulin as Determinants of Weight Loss on Diets Varying in Macronutrients and Dietary

Fibers-The POUNDS LOST Study. Nutrients 2019;11(3). https://doi.org/10.3390/nu11030586.

122. Gardner CD, Trepanowski JF, Del Gobbo LC, et al. Effect of Low-Fat vs Low-Carbohydrate Diet on 12-Month Weight Loss in Overweight Adults and the Association With Genotype Pattern or Insulin Secretion: The DIETFITS Randomized Clinical Trial. JAMA 2018;319(7):667–79.

123. Naude CE, Brand A, Schoonees A, et al. Low-carbohydrate versus balanced-carbohydrate diets for reducing weight and cardiovascular risk. Cochrane Database Syst Rev 2022;1:CD013334.

Preventive Nutrition
Heart Disease and Cancer

Connie J. Rogers, PhD, MPH[a], Kristina Petersen, PhD[b],
Penny M. Kris-Etherton, PhD, RD, FNLA, CLS[c],*

KEYWORDS

- Cardiovascular disease • Cancer • Healthy dietary patterns
- Dietary recommendations

KEY POINTS

- A healthy dietary pattern (that emphasizes a wide variety of plant foods and lean protein foods) is recommended for prevention of cardiovascular disease (CVD) and cancer.
- There is strong and consistent scientific evidence that a healthy dietary pattern significantly decreases risk of the major cardiovascular diseases and cancers.
- Optimal dietary adherence has the greatest benefits on CVD and cancer risk reduction; however, small increases in diet quality significantly reduce risk.
- A healthy dietary pattern can contribute significantly to reducing the massive global economic burden of CVD and cancer.

INTRODUCTION

From 1933 to 2018, diseases of the heart and malignant neoplasms were the top 2 causes of death in the United States.[1] Globally, from 1990 to 2017, the top 2 causes of mortality were cardiovascular diseases and cancers.[2] Most recent estimates indicate that cancer accounted for approximately 10 million deaths in 2020, more than any other cause.[3] The prevalence for both of these chronic diseases is continuing to increase along with a staggering economic burden of direct health care costs, direct nonhealth care costs, and indirect costs. The total global annual economic cost of cancer in 2010 was estimated at $1.16 trillion.[4] The annual direct and indirect cost of cardiovascular disease (CVD) in the United States from 2016 to 2017 was

C.J. Rogers and K. Petersen shared equally in the preparation of the article.
[a] Department of Nutritional Sciences, University of Georgia, 280 Dawson Hall, Athens, GA 30602, USA; [b] Department of Nutritional Sciences, Texas Tech University, 508 Human Sciences Building, Lubbock, TX 79409 USA; [c] Department of Nutritional Sciences, The Pennsylvania State University, 319 Chandlee Lab, University Park, PA 16802 USA
* Corresponding author. Department of Nutritional Sciences, Penn State University, 319 Chandlee Lab, University Park, PA 16802.
E-mail address: pmk3@psu.edu

approximately $363.4 billion.[5] Moreover, approximately $183 billion was spent in the United States on cancer-related health care in 2015, and this is projected to increase to $246 billion by 2030.[6]

Dietary exposures are implicated in the development of CVD and some cancers. However, it is now recognized that the totality of the diet has a greater effect on health outcomes than individual dietary components, including nutrients and foods. In alignment, dietary guidance in the United States and many other countries has shifted to focus on recommending dietary patterns that are characterized by high consumption of vegetables, fruits, whole grains, low-fat dairy, plant-based and lean protein foods, seafood, nuts and seeds, and plant oils. Healthy dietary patterns are also lower in red and processed meat, ultraprocessed foods, refined grains, and sugar-sweetened foods and beverages. Low/no to moderate consumption of alcohol also is a common feature of all healthy dietary patterns. These recommended dietary patterns are nutrient dense, meet all nutrient needs, and also are low in saturated fat, sodium, and added sugars. The purpose of this article is to summarize recent evidence on the relationship of diet quality as measured by adherence to healthy dietary patterns and CVD and cancer risk reduction.

The relationship between dietary patterns and risk of CVD, cancer, and cancer progression has been explored in 2 ways: (1) defining dietary patterns a priori based on a set of established criteria (eg, healthy eating index (HEI) or Mediterranean diet (MED) score), and (2) using statistical methods (eg, cluster analyses, factor analyses, principal component analyses) to evaluate dietary patterns in a population a posteriori. Numerous a priori dietary patterns based on either country-specific guidelines or chronic disease prevention guidelines have been examined in epidemiologic studies. Most dietary pattern scores contain component scores for fruits, vegetables, nuts and/or seeds, legumes, grains and meat; but some differ in other components including alcohol, dairy products, sodium and sugar-sweetened beverages. The results from systematic reviews and meta-analyses on dietary patterns and CVD and cancer will be summarized.

DIETARY PATTERNS AND CARDIOVASCULAR DISEASE RISK
Cardiovascular Disease

The 2020 Dietary Guidelines Advisory Committee (DGAC) concluded that strong and consistent evidence demonstrates that dietary patterns associated with decreased risk of CVD are characterized by higher consumption of vegetables, fruits, whole grains, low-fat dairy, and seafood, and lower intake of red and processed meat, refined grains, and sugar-sweetened foods and beverages.[7] In addition, regular intake of nuts and legumes and moderate intake of alcohol are also components of cardioprotective diets. The 2020 DGAC also concluded that randomized studies have shown that healthy dietary patterns exert clinically meaningful impact on cardiovascular risk factors, including blood lipids and blood pressure. Additionally, dietary patterns that are lower in saturated fat, cholesterol, and sodium, and higher in fiber, potassium, and unsaturated fats reduce CVD risk. Based on these conclusions, the evidence available for prevention of other chronic diseases, and the Dietary Reference Intakes, 3 US Department of Agriculture (USDA) Food Patterns were developed (Healthy US-Style Pattern, Healthy Mediterranean-Style Pattern, and the Healthy Vegetarian Pattern).[8] In addition, the Dietary Approaches to Stop Hypertension (DASH) Dietary Pattern, and the Mediterranean Dietary Pattern are recommended for CVD risk reduction.[9–11] The evidence for these dietary patterns and their relationship to CVD risk reduction will be summarized.

In a large prospective cohort study of women from the Nurses' Health Study (NHS) (n = 74,930) and the NHS II (n = 90,864) and men from the Health Professionals Follow-up Study (HPFS) (n = 43,339) compared with individuals in the lowest quintile of diet quality, those in the highest quintile had a lower risk of CVD (pooled hazard ratio [HR], 0.83; 95% confidence interval [CI], 0.79 to 0.86) (assessed by HEI-2015, which is based on the 2015 Dietary Guidelines for Americans).[12] Of note, a 25-percentile higher dietary score was associated with 10% to 20% lower risk of CVD (pooled HR, 0.80; 95% CI, 0.77 to 0.83). In an earlier analysis of the NHS and the HPFS, individuals who had the greatest improvement in diet quality assessed by the Alternative Healthy Eating Index (AHEI) had a 7% to 8% lower CVD risk in the subsequent 4-year period (HR, 0.92, 95% CI: 0.87 to 0.99, P-trend <.05).[13] In contrast, the authors reported an increase in CVD risk over 10 years with a 14% decrease in AHEI (95% CI: 2% to 27%).

Similar CVD benefits of adherence to the DASH dietary pattern have been reported. In the study by Morze and colleagues,[14] participants with the highest versus lowest DASH diet quality score had a reduced risk of incident CVD or mortality (RR 0.80, 95% CI 0.78 to 0.82). Likewise, in an umbrella review of 3 systematic reviews and meta-analyses of 15 prospective cohort studies (n = 942,140) and 4 systematic reviews and meta-analyses of controlled trials (n = 4414), the DASH dietary pattern was associated with decreased incident CVD (RR, 0.80 (0.76–0.85)).[15] In the controlled trials, the authors reported decreased systolic (MD, −5.2 mm Hg (95% CI, −7.0 to −3.4)) and diastolic (−2.60 mm Hg (−3.50 to −1.70)) blood pressure, total cholesterol (−0.20 mmol/L (−0.31 to −0.10)), and low-density lipoprotein (LDL) cholesterol (−0.10 mmol/L (−0.20 to −0.01)). Sotos-Prieto and colleagues[13] reported a decrease (16%) in DASH score was associated an 8% (95% CI: 2% to 15%) higher risk of CVD over the subsequent 20 years.

Two seminal clinical trials have reported marked beneficial effects of a Mediterranean-style diet on primary and secondary prevention of CVD. The Prevención con Dieta Mediterránea (PREDIMED) intervention trial conducted in Spain with 7477 participants at risk of CVD reported that CVD risk was reduced by 31% in participants consuming a Mediterranean diet with extra-virgin olive oil (50 g/d) and 28% in participants on a Mediterranean diet with mixed nuts (30 g/d) compared with the lower-fat control diet group after 4.8 years.[16]

The Lyon Diet Heart Study (conducted in France) evaluated a Mediterranean-type diet on the rate of recurrence after a first myocardial infarction (n = 605 participants). After 46 months of follow-up, the study was stopped early because of positive results. Participants following the Mediterranean-style diet had a 50% to 70% lower risk of recurrent heart disease, as measured by 3 different composite outcome measures: (1) cardiac deaths, nonfatal heart attacks; (2) the preceding plus unstable angina, stroke, heart failure, and pulmonary or peripheral embolism; and (3) all of these events plus those that required hospitalization.[17]

There have been 3 systematic reviews that evaluated the benefits of a Mediterranean-style diet on CVD risk, one of which was based on randomized controlled trials (RCTs) and two based on cohort studies. A recent Cochrane Review evaluated the effectiveness of a Mediterranean-style diet for the primary and secondary prevention of CVD compared with no intervention, minimal intervention, usual care, or another dietary intervention.[18] Based on 30 RCTs with 12,461 participants and 7 ongoing trials, the authors concluded that there is uncertainty about the effects of a Mediterranean-style diet on CVD, as well as risk factors in primary and secondary prevention studies.[18] However, 2 systematic reviews and meta-analyses of cohort studies reported benefits of a Mediterranean diet on CVD risk,[19,20] one of which was done in participants who had a history of CVD.[20] In the systematic review and meta-analysis of 29 articles conducted by Rosato and colleagues,[19] the RR for the highest versus the lowest category of the Mediterranean diet score was 0.81 (95% CI 0.74 to 0.88) for the 11 studies that considered unspecified CVD. In the systematic review and meta-analysis of 7 cohort studies with 37,879 participants who had a history of CVD,[20] the HR was 0.91 (95% CI; 0.82 to 1.01; n = 4) for cardiovascular mortality for each 2-unit increment in the Mediterranean diet adherence score. These results demonstrate that a Mediterranean diet may benefit individuals with a history of CVD; however, the findings await confirmation via RCTs. Nonetheless, on balance the evidence supports the conclusion that a Mediterranean diet decreases CVD risk.

Of note is that the Cochrane Review did report small benefits of a Mediterranean diet on 2 major CVD risk factors, elevated LDL cholesterol and blood pressure.[18] Some studies showed a possible small reduction in total cholesterol (−0.16 mmol/L, 95% CI -0.32 to 0.00), LDL cholesterol (−0.15 mmol/L, 95% CI -0.27 to −0.02), triglycerides (−0.09 mmol/L, 95% CI -0.16 to −0.01), and in systolic (−2.99 mm Hg , 95% CI -3.45 to −2.53) and diastolic blood pressure (−2.0 mm Hg, 95% CI -2.29 to −1.71). The blood pressure-lowering results agree with a recent systematic review and meta-analysis of 19 RCTs with 4137 participants and 16 observational studies with 59,001 participants that reported a reduction in systolic blood pressure and diastolic blood pressure of −1.4 mm Hg (95% CI: −2.40 to −0.39 mm Hg, P=.007) and −1.5 mm Hg (95% CI −2.74 to −0.32 mm Hg, P=.013), respectively, in response to a Mediterranean diet.[21]

Coronary Heart Disease

A meta-analysis of 12 prospective cohort studies including 409,780 participants from different countries reported an inverse association between a healthy dietary pattern and coronary heart disease (CHD) risk (RR = 0.80, 95% CI: 0.74 to 0.87).[22] Similar to the results reported for CVD, small differences in diet quality were associated with significantly lower risk of CHD. The analysis by Shan and colleagues,[12] described previously, reported the pooled HR for CHD per 25-percentile increase in dietary score (based on HEI-2015) was 0.78 (95% CI, 0.74 to 0.82). In a prospective cohort study by Sotos-Prieto and colleagues,[13] individuals in the highest quintile of 4-year change in diet quality (assessed by the AHEI) had a 12% lower CHD risk (95% CI 4% to 19%). In addition, over a 4-year period, participants with a 20-percentile increase in AHEI had a 6% lower CHD risk.[13] Similar to the results reported for CVD, an umbrella review of systematic reviews and meta-analyses of prospective cohort studies and controlled trials reported that a DASH dietary pattern was associated with decreased incident CHD (RR, 0.79 [0.71 to −0.88]).[15] In addition, a systematic review and meta-analysis of 11 observational studies reported that a Mediterranean dietary pattern was associated with a pooled RR for CHD and acute myocardial infarct risk (0.70 [95% CI 0.62 to 0.80]).[19]

Stroke

Based on a review of meta-analyses (n = of 87 mainly cohort studies), an ad hoc Working Group of the Italian Society of Human Nutrition (Italian Stroke Organization and the Stroke Prevention and Educational Awareness Diffusion) reported that there is strong evidence that a healthy dietary pattern, a DASH dietary pattern, and a Mediterranean dietary pattern all benefit stroke risk.[23] Similar to the studies for CVD and CHD, improvements in diet quality benefit stroke risk. In agreement, the analysis by Shan and colleagues[12] for stroke reported that the pooled HR 25-percentile increase in dietary score (based on HEI-2015) was 0.88 (95% CI, 0.81 to 0.96).

Most of the evidence for benefits of a healthy diet for reduced stroke risk is based on systematic reviews of DASH and Mediterranean-style dietary patterns. A systematic review and meta-analysis of 12 prospective cohort studies with 548,632 participants from the United States, Europe, and Asia reported that higher adherence versus lower adherence to the DASH diet was related to a reduced risk of stroke (RR 0.88, 95% CI 0.83 to 0.93). For each 4-point increment in DASH diet score, there was a total stroke risk reduction of 4% (RR 0.96, 95% CI 0.94 to 0.97).[24] In an umbrella review of systematic reviews and meta-analyses of prospective cohort studies and controlled trials, Chiavaroli and colleagues[15] reported that the DASH dietary pattern was associated with decreased stroke incidence (RR, 0.81 [0.72 to 0.92]). A systematic review and meta-analysis by Soltani and colleagues[25] evaluated the relationship between DASH diet adherence and the risk of stroke mortality in 2 cohorts with 193,036 participants. The HR was 0.97 (95% CI: 0.96 to 0.98) for each 5-point increase in the adherence to the DASH diet. Also, in the study by Sotos-Prieto and colleagues,[13] participants in the highest quintile for diet quality had a 15% lower stroke risk (95% CI, 3% to 26%). These authors also reported that a 20-percentile increase in the DASH diet score over a 4-year period was significantly associated with a 9% lower stroke risk.

In the systematic review and meta-analysis by Rosato and colleagues,[19] the RR was 0.82 (95% CI 0.73 to 0.92) for ischemic stroke (5 studies) and 1.01 (95% CI 0.74 to 1.37) for hemorrhagic stroke (4 studies).[19] The authors concluded that there was a benefit of a Mediterranean dietary pattern on ischemic stroke but not hemorrhagic stroke. Findings from PREDIMED demonstrated a reduction in the number of strokes with the Mediterranean diet intervention (HR 0.60, 95% CI 0.45 to 0.80).[16] In another meta-analysis of 20 prospective cohorts with 682,149 participants (that included unpublished results from the Singapore Chinese Health Study and the Seguimiento Universidad de Navarra [SUN] study) the RRs for each 4-point increment (which represented the highest vs the lowest quintiles of the MedDiet score) were reported.[26] There was a significant 16% (RR 0.84, 95% CI 0.81 to 0.88) lower risk of stroke for each 4-point increment in the MedDiet score for ischemic and hemorrhagic stroke. The Mediterranean dietary pattern was associated with lower risk of ischemic stroke (RR 0.86, 95% CI 0.81 to 0.91) and hemorrhagic stroke (RR 0.83, 95% CI 0.74 to 0.93).

Summary of Dietary Patterns and Cardiovascular Disease Research

The 2021 Dietary Guidance to Improve Cardiovascular Health from the American Heart Association recommends a healthy dietary pattern to promote optimal cardiovascular health.[11] Evidence from 3 large US cohorts (the Dietary Patterns Methods Project) reported a 14% to 28% lower CVD mortality in response to a high-quality versus a low-quality dietary pattern.[27] Higher dietary quality, regardless of the specific dietary pattern, is consistently associated with significantly decreased risk of CVD, CHD, and stroke. Likewise, higher dietary quality also benefits CVD risk factor status. These studies have consistently shown that small improvements in diet quality can meaningfully lower risk of CVD, CHD, and stroke. Importantly, there are benefits for primary prevention and secondary prevention, as well as for high-risk individuals.

DIETARY PATTERNS AND CANCER RISK, RECURRENCE AND MORTALITY

Diet is an established risk factor for several cancer types.[28] Individual nutrients and/or bioactive ingredients in food have been strongly associated with certain cancer types, for example, calcium and colorectal cancer (CRC).[28] The effectiveness of different dietary patterns in reducing cancer risk likely depends on the type of cancer, and other relevant risk factors such as family history, age, sex, body weight, physical activity, and smoking. However, multiple systematic reviews and meta-analyses, and the recommendations from the 2018 World Cancer Research Fund/American Institute for Cancer Research Third Expert Report[28] and the Scientific Report of the 2020 Dietary Guidelines Committee,[7] suggest that healthy dietary patterns may reduce the risk of several common cancer types including breast and CRC, and emerging data suggest a possible role of healthy dietary patterns in reducing several other cancer types.[7,28] Additionally, as cancer survival rates continue to improve, there is a need to identify dietary patterns that may prevent recurrence and mortality among cancer survivors. Understanding the relationship between dietary patterns and cancer risk and progression may result in clearer public health messages regarding beneficial nutritional strategies across the cancer prevention continuum.

Breast Cancer

Breast cancer represents the most common cancer in women[28] and leading cause of cancer death among women worldwide.[29] In 2020, there were approximately 2.3 million new breast cancer cases and 685,000 breast cancer deaths worldwide.[29] Thus, gaining a better understanding of the lifestyle factors that impact breast cancer risk and progression is an important public health issue that could impact the lives of millions of women.

A meta-analyses including 10 prospective cohort and 86 cross-sectional studies reported a decreased overall risk of cancer in those consuming a vegetarian or vegan diet (overall cancer RR = 0.92, 95% CI 0.87 to 0.98 and RR = 0.85, 95% CI 0.75 to 0.95), respectively.[30] However, no significant risk reduction specifically of breast cancer was observed in women consuming a vegetarian or vegan diet (breast cancer RR = 0.94, 95% CI 0.84 to 1.06).[30]

A systematic review including 6 cohort studies and 1 case-control study examined 12 different diet quality scores: 2 versions of the Dietary Inflammatory Index (DII), 4 versions of the Mediterranean diet score (MDS), the HEI, AHEI, DASH scores, and 3 versions of low-carbohydrate diet scores that differentiate between different sources of protein and fat on postmenopausal estrogen receptor-negative breast cancer risk. Of the 4 studies using MDS, 3 showed a significant inverse association with postmenopausal estrogen receptor-negative breast cancer; whereas no consistent association was observed with the other diet quality scores.[31]

A systematic review including 17 case-control and nested case-control studies evaluated dietary patterns using a priori and posteriori approaches. Six studies characterizing 5 dietary indices a priori including HEI, AHEI, Alternative Mediterranean Diet (aMed), MDS, and Healthy Nordic Food Index (HNFI), demonstrated a beneficial association between adherence to the HEI, AHEI, aMED, and MDS and breast cancer risk.[32] However, 3 studies evaluating diet quality using the MDS and 1 study evaluating diet quality using the HNFI found no association between adherence to these indices and breast cancer risk.[32] A systematic review including 5 cohort studies and 3 case-control studies examined the relationship between diet pattern using the DII and reported an increased risk of breast cancer with a high DII score (more inflammatory diet) (RR = 1.14, 95% CI 1.01 to 1.27).[33]

Determination of healthy and unhealthy dietary patterns a posteriori using a novel scoring matrix in alignment with the American Cancer Society (ACS) dietary guidelines identified 15 healthy and 10 unhealthy dietary patterns. A healthy dietary pattern was associated in 6 of 15 studies with a reduced risk and an unhealthy dietary pattern in 5 of 10 studies was associated with an increased risk of breast cancer. More specifically, consumption of vegetables was consistently associated with dietary patterns associated with reduced risk, whereas saturated fat and red and processed meats were consistently found in patterns associated with increased breast cancer risk.[32]

Two additional systematic reviews or meta-analyses have examined the relationship between healthy or unhealthy dietary patterns a posteriori and breast cancer risk. Albuquerque and colleagues evaluated data from 11 cohort and 15 case-control studies and found that a "vegetable, fruit, fish and soy" pattern and a "Mediterranean" pattern were associated with a decreased risk and a "Western" pattern and a "drinker" pattern increased breast risk.[34] A "Western" pattern also significantly increased breast cancer risk (RR = 1.14, 95% CI 1.02 to 1.28) and a "prudent" pattern decreased breast cancer risk (RR = 0.82, 95% CI 0.75 to 0.89) in a meta-analyses including 14 cohort and 18 case-control studies.[35] Furthermore, every category of alcohol consumption, from light to heavy drinking, was associated with an increased risk of breast cancer (RR = 1.04, 95% CI 1.01 to 1.07 for light), (RR = 1.23, 95% CI 1.19 to 1.28 for moderate), (RR = 1.61, 95% CI 1.33, 1.94 for heavy drinking) in a meta-analysis including 118 studies.[36]

Several RCTs have evaluated dietary patterns on breast cancer risk and mortality. The Women's Health Initiative Dietary Modification (DM) trial evaluated whether a low-fat dietary pattern reduced the risk of breast cancer (CRC and CHD risk also assessed) in 48,835 postmenopausal women. Participants were randomly assigned to a low-fat dietary pattern intervention group (reduce fat intake from approximately 35% to 20% of total energy, in conjunction with increasing vegetables and fruit to 5 servings/d and grains to 6 servings/d) or to a usual-diet comparison group, during a 5-year period. No differences in breast cancer risk were observed during the 8.5-year intervention period between the intervention and control group.[37] However, in women with higher baseline fat intake, breast cancer risk during the intervention was lower compared with the during postintervention follow-up (HR = 0.76, 95% CI 0.62-0.92 vs HR = 1.11, 95% CI 0.84-1.4). Furthermore, during a 19.6-year median follow-up period, a significant reduction in breast-cancer related mortality (HR = 0.84, 95% CI 0.74-0.96) was observed in the intervention group.[38,39]

Several other studies have examined the relationship between dietary patterns and breast cancer recurrence and mortality. A meta-analyses including 83 studies (including RCTs, cohort, and case-control studies) and an overall population of 2,130,753 subjects found that the highest adherence score to a Mediterranean diet was inversely associated with a lower risk of overall cancer mortality (RR = 0.86, 95% CI 0.81-0.91, 15 cohort studies), but no effect of diet was observed in 1 RCT.[40] However, when examining the association between the adherence to the highest Mediterranean diet category and cancer mortality among cancer survivors specifically, no association was observed (RR = 0.95, 95% CI 0.82-1.12, 4 studies). With respect to an association between the adherence to the highest Mediterranean diet category and risk of mortality from breast cancer, a beneficial effect was observed in 1 RCT (RR = 0.43, 95% CI 0.21-0.88), and in pooled data from 16 observational studies (RR = 0.92, 95% CI 0.89-0.96), 7 cohort studies (RR = 0.94, 95% CI 0.90-0.99), and 9 case-control studies (RR = 0.89, 95% CI 0.85-0.94).[40]

One systematic review including 7 studies (dietary patterns were defined a priori in 4 and a posteriori in 3) reported an association between a healthy dietary pattern and reduced risk of breast cancer mortality in 2 of the 7 studies. In both of these studies, overall dietary intake was assessed a priori using the HEI-2005 (HR = 0.12, 95% CI 0.02-0.99) and DII (HR = 0.75, 95% CI 0.57-0.99).[41] An additional systematic review including 2 RCTs (same trials referenced previously[38,39]) and 16 cohort studies assessed dietary patterns using a priori and a posteriori methods. Dietary indices were examined after a breast cancer diagnosis from participants in the Health, Eating, Activity, and Lifestyle (HEAL) study;[42] Women's Health Initiative's Dietary Modification Trial and Observational Study (WHI);[43] NHS;[44] and the Cancer Prevention Study II Nutrition Cohort (CPS-II).[45] The HEI-2005, the AHEI, the World Cancer Research Fund, and the American Institute for Cancer Research (WCRF/AIRC) dietary guidelines adherence score and the ACS diet-specific recommendations for cancer prevention, the recommended food score (RFS), the Diet Quality Index-Revised (DQIR), the DASH diet, the HNFI, and the aMed diet were the indices used to assess dietary patterns/quality. Most studies demonstrated no association between dietary pattern and breast cancer mortality, although 2 studies reported a negative association between breast cancer mortality and higher adherence to the HEI-2005 index.[46] Closer adherence to HEA-2005, DASH, AHEI, and ACS dietary patterns was also associated with a lower risk of death from other causes and overall mortality in studies using data from all 4 prospective cohorts (HEAL, WHI, NHS, and CPS-II).[46] When a posteriori diet patterns were evaluated, adherence to a high-quality diet, low-fat diet, or prudent diet after diagnosis was associated with a decreased risk of all-cause mortality but not breast cancer-specific mortality. Moreover, adherence to a Western diet before and after diagnosis was associated with higher overall mortality risk and death from other causes.[46]

Colorectal Cancer

CRC is the third most common cancer worldwide, especially in developed countries where an estimated 60% of all cases occur.[3,28] Many studies have demonstrated that plant phytochemicals and dietary fiber have a strong chemopreventive role in the onset of CRC.[47] Thus, exploring dietary patterns that may prevent the risk and progression of CRC has important public health implications.

Numerous dietary pattern indices, including HEI, AHEI, DASH, MED, Dietary Inflammatory Index (DII), WCRF/AICR, HNFI, and vegetarian, have been used to evaluate the association between dietary patterns and CRC. Four systematic reviews and/or meta-analyses evaluated MED or HEI CRC risk, and 1 narrative review examined MED only on CRC risk. All 5 reviews reported that greater index scores or greater adherence to a healthy diet pattern was associated with lower risk of developing CRC. Specifically, Donovan and colleagues reported a decreased risk of CRC in 3 out of 3 case-control studies and 3 out of 5 cohort studies with greater MDS.[48] A meta-analyses including 11 studies found that the highest adherence score to a Mediterranean diet was inversely associated with a lower risk CRC (RR = 0.82, 95% CI 0.75-0.88).[40] In a systematic review including 7 cohort and 5 case-control studies, 5 studies examined the MDS, and 4 examined the HEI comparing highest to lowest score groups. A higher MDS was associated with an 8% to 54% lower CRC risk, and higher HEI scores were associated with a 20% to 56% lower CRC risk.[49] A meta-analyses including 28 cohort and 21 case-control studies demonstrated that healthy dietary patterns assessed with a higher MED and HEI, as well as DASH, WCRF/AICR and vegetarian diet decreased CRC risk.[50] For the MED dietary pattern score, the 3 cohort studies found an 11% to 28% lower risk of CRC, and the 3 case-control studies found higher risk reductions ranging from 13% to 54% lower odds of CRC, comparing the highest to the lowest score category.[50]

Four systematic reviews or meta-analyses examined the relationship between DII and CRC risk.

Findings were consistent across all studies, with a higher DII associated with increased risk of CRC. Tabung and colleagues reported that 3 case-control studies using the DII reported higher OR from 1.55 to 2.16 with higher (more proinflammatory) scores, and 4 cohort studies reported 16% to 40% higher risk of CRC with higher DII.[50] Two additional meta-analyses reported an increase risk of CRC with higher DII score (high DII, RR = 1.40, 95% CI 1.26-1.55[51] and RR = 1.43, 95% CI, 1.26-1.62).[52]

Three systematic reviews or meta-analyses examined the relationship between a posteriori dietary patterns and CRC risk. One study found that a healthy pattern was associated with decreased risk of CRC in 10 out of 12 case-control studies and in 4 out of 10 cohort studies. Additionally, an unhealthy pattern was associated with increased risk in 11 out of 13 case-control studies and 6 out of 11 cohort studies.[50] The major food groups in the healthy pattern included fruits and vegetables, nuts and legumes, milk and other dairy products, and some fish/seafood and poultry, while the main constituents of the unhealthy dietary pattern included red and processed meat, sugar-sweetened beverages, refined grains, desserts, and potatoes. In support of these data, the AICR Continuous Update Project concludes that there is strong evidence linking consumption of whole grains and dietary fiber to lowered risk of CRC.[28] Two additional studies found that Western and drinker dietary patterns increased risk of CRC (RR = 1.25, 95% CI, 1.11-1.40 and RR = 1.19, 95% CI, 0.99-1.43, respectively), while a prudent pattern decreased risk (RR = 0.81, 95% CI, 0.73-0.91).[53,54] Furthermore, moderate and heavy drinking, but not light drinking, was associated with an increased risk of CRC (moderate drinking, RR = 1.17, 95% CI, 1.11-1.24 and heavy drinking, RR = 1.44, 95% CI 1.25-1.65) in a meta-analysis including 66 studies.[36]

Despite a consistent pattern among studies with a healthier diet pattern associated with lower risk of CRC, findings differed by sex and anatomic subsite. Some associations were stronger in men than women. Among the studies that reported results by subsite, more studies observed a significant relationship for colon cancer than rectal cancer.

Four systematic reviews and meta-analyses have explored the association between a priori and a posteriori dietary patterns and CRC mortality. The results are mixed with respect to the association between a priori dietary patterns, with 2 studies demonstrating a beneficial effect of adherence to the mMDS and/or the HNFI postcancer diagnosis on overall mortality[46,55] and 2 demonstrating no association between adherence to the aHEI, DASH, or aMED score after a cancer diagnosis, and mortality in CRC survivors.[56,57] Four studies found no association between adherence to a prudent diet[57-60]; however, a Western diet or a diet high in red and processed meats was associated with a greater risk of mortality in 5 studies.[57-61]

OTHER CANCER TYPES

The relationship between dietary patterns and other cancer types including lung, prostate and pancreatic cancers has been explored in fewer studies. Based on recommendations in the 2020 DGAC report and the 2018 WCRF/AICR report, there is limited evidence suggesting that dietary patterns containing more frequent servings of vegetables, fruits, seafood, grains and cereals, legumes, and lean vs higher fat meats and lower fat or nonfat dairy products may be associated with lower risk of lung cancer, primarily among former smokers and current smokers.[7] Furthermore, there is limited evidence suggesting no relationship between dietary patterns and risk of prostate and pancreatic cancer.

SUMMARY OF DIETARY PATTERNS AND CANCER RESEARCH

In summary, the 2018 World Cancer Research Fund/American Institute for Cancer Research Third Expert Report[28] and the Scientific Report of the 2020 Dietary Guidelines Advisory Committee[7] concluded that a moderate level of evidence exists demonstrating that healthy dietary patterns may reduce the risk of breast cancer and CRC. Results from recent systematic reviews and meta-analyses support this conclusion. Alcohol was not consistently part of the patterns found to be significantly associated with lower breast cancer or CRC risk, and in most cases, it was part of cases associated with increased risk. Emerging data suggest that healthy dietary patterns may also reduce breast cancer and CRC recurrence and mortality. However, the data are limited; thus, additional prospective cohort studies and RCTs are needed to determine if an association between any dietary pattern and breast cancer and/or CRC mortality exists. Limited data are available to make conclusions regarding adherence to a healthy dietary pattern and the risk and mortality from any other cancer type.

CONCLUDING REMARKS: DIETARY PATTERNS, CARDIOVASCULAR DISEASE AND CANCER RISK

Substantial consistency is observed in dietary risk factors for CVD and cancer. In the United States in 2019, 11.7% of CVD deaths and 1.4% of cancer deaths were attributable to dietary risk factors.[62] Dietary risks associated with CVD and cancer deaths included low intake of whole grains, fruit, fiber and vegetables, and high intake of red and processed meats and sodium.

Higher diet quality is associated with similar lowering of the relative risk of CVD and cancer. In a recent systematic review and meta-analysis of 113 cohort studies including 3,277,684 participants, higher diet quality was associated with lower relative risk of CVD incidence or mortality (RR 0.80, 95% CI 0.78-0.82) and cancer incidence or mortality (RR 0.86, 95% CI 0.84–0.89). In addition, in cancer survivors, the highest diet quality was associated with lower risk of all-cause (RR 0.83, 95% CI 0.77-0.88) and cancer mortality (RR 0.82, 95% CI 0.75-0.89).[14] Thus, higher diet quality evaluated by the HEI, AHEI and DASH indices significantly lowers the risk of CVD and cancer.

In alignment, there are many commonalities in the dietary recommendations for prevention of CVD and cancer. **Table 1** summarizes dietary recommendations issued for general health and chronic disease prevention as well as guidelines for prevention of CVD and cancer. The guidelines consistently recommend high intakes of vegetables, fruits, whole grains, legumes, nuts, and seeds, and lower intakes of sources of saturated fat, added sugar, and sodium. In addition, all of these guidelines recommend limiting alcohol intake. **Fig. 1** illustrates commonalities among recommended healthy dietary patterns.

In conclusion, CVD and cancer are leading causes of death and disability globally and in the United States. Despite differences in the etiology, diet-related risk factors for CVD and cancer are remarkably similar. Strong and consistent evidence shows higher diet quality, assessed by a priori defined indices, is associated with lower risk of CVD and cancer. Dietary guidelines for prevention of CVD and cancer recommend a diet rich in fruits, vegetables, whole grains, legumes, nuts and seeds. Red and processed meats, added sugars, sodium, and alcohol should be limited. Population level intervention to improve diet quality will have substantial public health benefit and may meaningfully lower the incidence of CVD and cancer.

Table 1
Dietary recommendation for general health and prevention of cardiovascular disease and cancer

Recommendations	General Health & Chronic Disease Prevention — Dietary Guidelines for Americans 2020–2025[8] (2000 kcal/d)			CVD Prevention		Cancer Prevention
	Healthy US-Style Dietary Pattern	Healthy Mediterranean-Style Dietary Pattern	Healthy Vegetarian Dietary Pattern	American Heart Association[11] — AHA 2021 Dietary Guidance to Improve Cardiovascular Health	National Lipid Association[9] — Nutrition Recommendations for Management of Dyslipidemia	World Cancer Research Fund International/American Institute for Cancer Research[63] — Recommendations for Cancer Prevention
Vegetables (cup/d)	2 ½	2 ½	2 ½	Eat plenty of fruits and vegetables, choose a wide variety.	Follow a healthy dietary pattern, including an emphasis on a variety of plant foods and lean sources of protein, for example, DASH, USDA (healthy US-style), AHA, Mediterranean style, and vegetarian/vegan	Eat a diet rich in whole grains, vegetables, fruits and beans • Consume a diet that provides ≥ 30 g/d of fiber from food • Include foods containing wholegrains, nonstarchy vegetables, fruit and pulses (legumes) such as beans and lentils in most meals • Eat a diet high in all types of plant foods including at least 5 portions or servings (at least 400g or 15 ounces in total) of a variety of nonstarchy vegetables and fruit every day • If you eat starchy roots and tubers as staple foods, eat nonstarchy vegetables, fruit and pulses (legumes) regularly too if possible
Dark-Green Vegetables (cups/week)	1 ½	1 ½	1 ½			
Red & Orange Vegetables (cups/week)	5 ½	5 ½	5 ½			
Beans, Peas, Lentils (cups/week)	1 ½	1 ½	1 ½			
Starchy Vegetables (cups/week)	5	5	5			
Other Vegetables (cups/week)	4	4	4			
Fruit (cups/d)	2	2 ½	2			
Grains (ounces/d)	6	6	6 ½			
Whole Grains (ounces/d)	≥3	3	3 ½	Choose foods mainly with whole grains rather than refined grains		
Refined Grains (ounces/d)	<3	3	3			
Dairy (cups/d)	3	2	3	Choose healthy surces of protein mostly protein from plants (legumes and nuts) Fish and seafood Low-fat or fat-free dairy products instead of full-fat dairy products		
Protein Foods (ounces/day)	5 ½	6 ½	3 ½			
	26	26	3 (eggs)			

(continued on next page)

Table 1 (continued)

Recommendations	General Health & Chronic Disease Prevention			CVD Prevention		Cancer Prevention
	Dietary Guidelines for Americans 2020-2025[8]			American Heart Association[11]	National Lipid Association[9]	World Cancer Research Fund International/American Institute for Cancer Research[63]
	Healthy US-Style Dietary Pattern	Healthy Mediterranean-Style Dietary Pattern	Healthy Vegetarian Dietary Pattern	AHA 2021 Dietary Guidance to Improve Cardiovascular Health	Nutrition Recommendations for Management of Dyslipidemia	Recommendations for Cancer Prevention
	(2000 kcal/d)					
Meats, Poultry, Eggs (ounces/week)				If meat or poultry are desired, choose lean cuts and avoid processed forms		Limit consumption of red and processed meat • If you eat red meat, limit consumption to no more than about 3 portions per week. Three portions are equivalent to about 350–500 g (about 12–18 ounces) cooked weight • Consume very little, if any, processed meat
Seafood (ounces/week)	8	15	6			
Nuts, Seeds, Soy Products (ounces/week)	5	5	8 Soy products 7 Nuts and seeds			
Beans, Peas, Lentils (cups/week)			6			
Oils (g/d)	27	27	27	Use liquid plant oils rather than tropical oils (coconut, palm, and palm kernel), animal fats (eg, butter and lard), and partially hydrogenated fats		
Limit on Calories for Other Uses (kcal/d)	240	240	250	Choose minimally processed foods instead of ultraprocessed foods		Limit consumption of fast foods and other processed foods high in fat, starches, or sugars • Limit consumption of processed foods high in fat, starches or sugars – including fast foods; many preprepared dishes, snacks, bakery foods, and desserts; and confectionery (candy)
Limit on Calories for Other Uses (% kcal/d)	12	12	13			

Saturated Fat (% kcal/d)	<10	-	<7	-
Added Sugars (% kcal/d)	<10	Minimize intake of beverages and foods with added sugars	<10 (avoid if triglycerides >500 mg/dL)	Limit consumption of sugar sweetened drinks
Sodium (mg/d)	<2300	Choose and prepare foods with little or no salt	<2300	-
Dietary Cholesterol (mg/d)	No recommendation (diets have <300 mg/d)	-	<200	-
Fiber (g/d)	28	-	5–10 (viscous)	≥ 30 g/d
Plant Sterols and Stanols (g/d)	-	-	~2	-
Alcohol	If you choose to drink alcohol, ≤2 drinks/d for men and ≤ 1 drink/day for women.	If you do not drink alcohol, do not start; if you choose to drink alcohol, limit intake	For adults who choose to consume alcohol, to do so in moderation. If triglycerides are very high (≥500 mg/dL), complete abstinence of alcohol is recommended	Limit alcohol consumption • For cancer prevention, it is best not to drink alcohol • If you do consume alcoholic drinks, do not exceed national guidelines

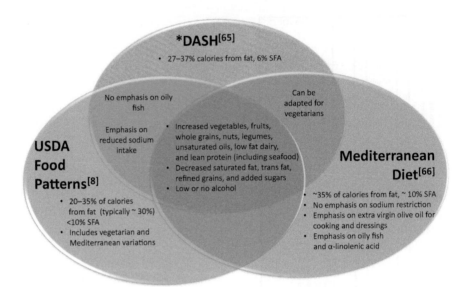

Fig. 1. Venn diagram of recommended dietary patterns illustrating shared characteristics. *The original DASH diet is 27% calories from fat with modifications being substitutions of calories from carbohydrates with unsaturated fat or protein (with permission from[64]). DASH dietary pattern,[65] USDA food pattern,[8] and Mediterranean diet.[66]

CLINICS CARE POINTS

- CVD and cancer are 2 leading causes of death globally.
- The totality of the diet has a greater effect on CVD and cancer outcomes than individual dietary components.
- The guidance in the United States and many other countries has shifted to focus on recommending dietary patterns that are characterized by high consumption of vegetables, fruits, whole grains, low-fat dairy, plant-based and lean protein foods, seafood, nuts and seeds, and plant oils and are lower in red and processed meat, ultraprocessed foods, refined grains, and sugar-sweetened foods and beverages, and consumption of alcohol.
- Higher dietary quality, regardless of the specific dietary pattern, is consistently associated with significantly decreased risk of CVD, CHD, stroke, breast cancer, and CRC.
- A healthy dietary pattern throughout the lifespan is an important lifestyle factor to prevent risk, progression and mortality from CVD and cancer.

DISCLOSURE

The authors have nothing to disclose.

REFERENCES

1. Harding MC, Sloan CD, Merrill RM, et al. Transitions from heart disease to cancer as the leading cause of death in US States, 1999-2016. Prev Chronic Dis 2018;15: E158.

2. Ritchie H, Roser M. Causes of death. 2019. https://ourworldindata.org/causes-of-death.

3. Ferlay J, Colombet M, Soerjomataram I, et al. Cancer statistics for the year 2020: An overview. Int J Cancer April 5 2021 (online ahead of print).

4. The International Agency for Research on Cancer. World cancer report: cancer research for cancer prevention. Lyon (France): International Agency for Research on Cancer; 2020.

5. Virani SS, Alonso A, Aparicio HJ, et al. Heart disease and stroke statistics-2021 update: a report from the American Heart Association. Circulation 2021;143(8): e254–743.

6. Mariotto AB, Enewold L, Zhao J, et al. Medical care costs associated with cancer survivorship in the United States. Cancer Epidemiol Biomarkers Prev 2020;29(7): 1304–12.

7. Dietary Guidelines Advisory Committee. Scientific Report of the 2020 Dietary Guidelines Advisory Committee advisory report to the secretary of agriculture and the secretary of health and human services. Washington, DC: U.S. Department of Agriculture, Agricultural Research Service; 2020.

8. U.S. Department of Agriculture and U.S. Department of Health and Human Services, Dietary Guidelines for Americans 2020–2025. 9th Edition. 2020: Washington, DC.

9. Jacobson TA, Maki KC, Orringer CE, et al. National lipid association recommendations for patient-centered management of dyslipidemia: Part 2. J Clin Lipidol 2015;9(6 Suppl):S1–122.e1.

10. Arnett DK, Blumenthal RS, Albert MA, et al. 2019 ACC/AHA guideline on the primary prevention of cardiovascular disease: a report of the American College of Cardiology/American Heart Association task force on clinical practice guidelines. Circulation 2019;140(11):e596–646.

11. Lichtenstein AH, Appel LJ, Vadiveloo M, et al. 2021 Dietary guidance to improve cardiovascular health: a scientific statement from the American Heart Association. Circulation 2021;144(23):e472–87.

12. Shan Z, Baden MY, Bhupathiraju SN, et al. Association between healthy eating patterns and risk of cardiovascular disease. JAMA Intern Med 2020;180(8): 1090–100.

13. Sotos-Prieto M, Bhupathiraju SN, Mattei J, et al. Changes in diet quality scores and risk of cardiovascular disease among US men and women. Circulation 2015;132(23):2212–9.

14. Morze J, Danielewicz A, Hoffmann G, et al. Diet quality as assessed by the healthy eating index, alternate healthy eating index, dietary approaches to stop hypertension score, and health outcomes: a second update of a systematic review and meta-analysis of cohort studies. J Acad Nutr Diet 2020;120(12): 1998–2031.e15.

15. Chiavaroli L, Viguiliouk E, Nishi SK, et al. DASH dietary pattern and cardiometabolic outcomes: an umbrella review of systematic reviews and meta-analyses. Nutrients 2019;11(2):338.

16. Estruch R, Ros E, Salas-Salvado J, et al. Primary prevention of cardiovascular disease with a mediterranean diet supplemented with extra-virgin olive oil or nuts. N Engl J Med 2018;378(25):e34.

17. de Lorgeril M, Salen P, Martin JL, et al. Mediterranean diet, traditional risk factors, and the rate of cardiovascular complications after myocardial infarction: final report of the Lyon Diet Heart Study. Circulation 1999;99(6):779–85.

18. Rees K, Takeda A, Martin N, et al. Mediterranean-style diet for the primary and secondary prevention of cardiovascular disease. Cochrane Database Syst Rev 2019;(3):CD009825.

19. Rosato V, Temple NJ, La Vecchiac C, et al. Mediterranean diet and cardiovascular disease: a systematic review and meta-analysis of observational studies. Eur J Nutr 2019;58(1):173–91.

20. Tang C, Wang X, Qin LQ, et al. Mediterranean diet and mortality in people with cardiovascular disease: a meta-analysis of prospective cohort studies. Nutrients 2021;13(8):2623.

21. Cowell OR, Mistry N, Deighton K, et al. Effects of a Mediterranean diet on blood pressure: a systematic review and meta-analysis of randomized controlled trials and observational studies. J Hypertens 2021;39(4):729–39.

22. Hou L, Li F, Wang Y, et al. Association between dietary patterns and coronary heart disease: a meta-analysis of prospective cohort studies. Int J Clin Exp Med 2015;8(1):781–90.

23. Iacoviello L, Bonaccio M, Cairella G, et al. Diet and primary prevention of stroke: systematic review and dietary recommendations by the ad hoc Working Group of the Italian Society of Human Nutrition. Nutr Metab Cardiovasc Dis 2018;28(4):309–34.

24. Feng Q, Fan S, Wu Y, et al. Adherence to the dietary approaches to stop hypertension diet and risk of stroke: a meta-analysis of prospective studies. Medicine (Baltimore) 2018;97(38):e12450.

25. Soltani S, Arablou T, Jayedi A, et al. Adherence to the dietary approaches to stop hypertension (DASH) diet in relation to all-cause and cause-specific mortality: a systematic review and dose-response meta-analysis of prospective cohort studies. Nutr J 2020;19(1):37.

26. Chen GC, Neelakantan N, Martin-Calvo N, et al. Adherence to the Mediterranean diet and risk of stroke and stroke subtypes. Eur J Epidemiol 2019;34(4):337–49.

27. Liese AD, Kreb-Smith SM, Subar AF, et al. The dietary patterns methods project: synthesis of findings across cohorts and relevance to dietary guidance. J Nutr 2015;145(3):393–402.

28. World Cancer Research Fund/ American Institute for Cancer Research. Diet, nutrition, physical activity and cancer: a global perspective. Continuous Update Project Expert Report; 2018.

29. Lei S, Zheng R, Zhang S, et al. Global patterns of breast cancer incidence and mortality: a population-based cancer registry data analysis from 2000 to 2020. Cancer Commun (Lond) 2021;41(11):1183–94.

30. Dinu M, Abbate R, Gensini GF, et al. Vegetarian, vegan diets and multiple health outcomes: a systematic review with meta-analysis of observational studies. Crit Rev Food Sci Nutr 2017;57(17):3640–9.

31. Du M, Liu SH, Mitchell C, et al. Associations between diet quality scores and risk of postmenopausal estrogen receptor-negative breast cancer: a systematic review. J Nutr 2018;148(1):100–8.

32. Dandamudi A, Tommie J, Nommsen-Rivers L, et al. Dietary patterns and breast cancer risk: a systematic review. Anticancer Res 2018;38(6):3209–22.

33. Zahedi H, Djalalinia S, Sadeghi O, et al. Dietary inflammatory potential score and risk of breast cancer: systematic review and meta-analysis. Clin Breast Cancer 2018;18(4):e561–70.

34. Albuquerque RC, Baltar VT, Marchioni DM. Breast cancer and dietary patterns: a systematic review. Nutr Rev 2014;72(1):1–17.

35. Xiao Y, Xia J, Li L, et al. Associations between dietary patterns and the risk of breast cancer: a systematic review and meta-analysis of observational studies. Breast Cancer Res 2019;21(1):16.
36. Bagnardi V, Rota M, Botteri E, et al. Alcohol consumption and site-specific cancer risk: a comprehensive dose-response meta-analysis. Br J Cancer 2015;112(3):580–93.
37. Thomson CA, Van Horn L, Caan BJ, et al. Cancer incidence and mortality during the intervention and postintervention periods of the Women's Health Initiative dietary modification trial. Cancer Epidemiol Biomarkers Prev 2014;23(12):2924–35.
38. Prentice RL, Aragaki AK, Howard BV, et al. Low-fat dietary pattern among postmenopausal women influences long-term cancer, cardiovascular disease, and diabetes outcomes. J Nutr 2019;149(9):1565–74.
39. Chlebowski RT, Aragaki AK, Anderson JL, et al. Dietary modification and breast cancer mortality: long-term follow-up of the women's health initiative randomized trial. J Clin Oncol 2020;38(13):1419–28.
40. Schwingshackl L, Schwedhelm C, Galbete C, et al. Adherence to Mediterranean diet and risk of cancer: an updated systematic review and meta-analysis. Nutrients 2017;9(10).
41. Terranova CO, Protani MM, Reeves MM. Overall dietary intake and prognosis after breast cancer: a systematic review. Nutr Cancer 2018;70(2):153–63.
42. George SM, Irwin ML, Smith AW, et al. Postdiagnosis diet quality, the combination of diet quality and recreational physical activity, and prognosis after early-stage breast cancer. Cancer Causes Control 2011;22(4):589–98.
43. George SM, Ballard-Barbash R, Shikany JM, et al. Better postdiagnosis diet quality is associated with reduced risk of death among postmenopausal women with invasive breast cancer in the women's health initiative. Cancer Epidemiol Biomarkers Prev 2014;23(4):575–83.
44. Kim EH, Willett WC, Fung T, et al. Diet quality indices and postmenopausal breast cancer survival. Nutr Cancer 2011;63(3):381–8.
45. McCullough ML, Gapstur SM, Shah R, et al. Pre- and postdiagnostic diet in relation to mortality among breast cancer survivors in the CPS-II Nutrition Cohort. Cancer Causes Control 2016;27(11):1303–14.
46. Jochems SHJ, Van Osch FHM, Bryan RT, et al. Impact of dietary patterns and the main food groups on mortality and recurrence in cancer survivors: a systematic review of current epidemiological literature. BMJ Open 2018;8(2):e014530.
47. Song M, Chan AT, Sun J. Influence of the gut microbiome, diet, and environment on risk of colorectal cancer. Gastroenterology 2020;158(2):322–40.
48. Donovan MG, Selmin OI, Doetschman TC, et al. Mediterranean diet: prevention of colorectal cancer. Front Nutr 2017;4:59.
49. Steck SE, Guinter M, Zheng J, et al. Index-based dietary patterns and colorectal cancer risk: a systematic review. Adv Nutr 2015;6(6):763–73.
50. Tabung FK, Brown LS, Fung TT. Dietary patterns and colorectal cancer risk: a review of 17 years of evidence (2000-2016). Curr Colorectal Cancer Rep 2017;13(6):440–54.
51. Shivappa N, Godos J, Hebert JR, et al. Dietary inflammatory index and colorectal cancer risk-a meta-analysis. Nutrients 2017;9(9):1043.
52. Fan Y, Jin X, Man C, et al. Meta-analysis of the association between the inflammatory potential of diet and colorectal cancer risk. Oncotarget 2017;8(35):59592–600.

53. Fardet A, Druesne-Pecollo N, Touvier M, et al. Do alcoholic beverages, obesity and other nutritional factors modify the risk of familial colorectal cancer? A systematic review. Crit Rev Oncol Hematol 2017;119:94–112.

54. Garcia-Larsen V, Morton V, Norat T, et al. Dietary patterns derived from principal component analysis (PCA) and risk of colorectal cancer: a systematic review and meta-analysis. Eur J Clin Nutr 2019;73(3):366–86.

55. Ratjen I, Schafmayer C, di Giuseppe R, et al. Postdiagnostic Mediterranean and healthy Nordic dietary patterns are inversely associated with all-cause mortality in long-term colorectal cancer survivors. J Nutr 2017;147(4):636–44.

56. Pelser C, Arem H, Pfeiffer RM, et al. Prediagnostic lifestyle factors and survival after colon and rectal cancer diagnosis in the National Institutes of Health (NIH)-AARP Diet and Health Study. Cancer 2014;120(10):1540–7.

57. Fung TT, Kashambwa R, Sato K, et al. Post diagnosis diet quality and colorectal cancer survival in women. PLoS One 2014;9(12):e115377.

58. Meyerhardt JA, Niedzwiecki D, Hollis D, et al. Association of dietary patterns with cancer recurrence and survival in patients with stage III colon cancer. JAMA 2007;298(7):754–64.

59. Zhu Y, Wu H, Wang PP, et al. Dietary patterns and colorectal cancer recurrence and survival: a cohort study. BMJ Open 2013;3(2).

60. Romaguera D, Ward H, Wark PA, et al. Pre-diagnostic concordance with the WCRF/AICR guidelines and survival in European colorectal cancer patients: a cohort study. BMC Med 2015;13:107.

61. Carr PR, Jansen L, Walter V, et al. Associations of red and processed meat with survival after colorectal cancer and differences according to timing of dietary assessment. Am J Clin Nutr 2016;103(1):192–200.

62. Institute for Health Metrics and Evaluation (IHME). GBD compare data visualization 2020. Available at: http://vizhub.healthdata.org/gbd-compare. Accessed April, 24, 2022.

63. Wild CP, Wiederpass E, Stewart BW, editors. World Cancer Report: cancer research for cancer prevention. Lyon (France): International Agency for Research on Cancer; 2020.

64. Skulus-Ray AC, Richter C, Cummings D. Dietary patterns for the prevention and treatment of cardiovascular disease. In: Ballantyne CM, editor. Clinical lipidology: a companion to Braunwald's heart disease. San Diego (CA): Elsevier Publishers; 2022.

65. NHLBI. 2021. Available at: https://www.nhlbi.nih.gov/education/dash-eating-plan. Accessed May 15, 2022.

66. Oldways. Oldways Mediterranean diet pyramid. Available at: https://oldwayspt.org/resources/oldways-mediterranean-diet-pyramid. Accessed May 15, 2022.

How Physicians Can Assess and Address Dietary Behaviors to Reduce Chronic Disease Risk

Caitlin A. Hildebrand, MD, MPH[a,b], David B. Gaviria, MPH, RD[a,b],
Carmen D. Samuel-Hodge, RD, PhD[a,b],
Alice S. Ammerman, DrPH[a,b], Thomas C. Keyserling, MD, MPH[a,c],*

KEYWORDS

- Dietary assessment • Dietary screening • Registered dietitian referral
- Team-based nutrition care • Eating disorder screening

KEY POINTS

- Diet is a major risk factor for many chronic diseases, and primary care providers (PCPs) have an important role in nutrition care for patients.
- Dietary assessment is an essential skill for PCPs and one that can be accomplished through the use of brief dietary assessment and counseling strategies.
- For patients who would benefit from comprehensive dietary counseling, registered dietitians are a valuable resource.
- Screening for eating disorders is an essential skill that can be accomplished through brief screening questionnaires.

INTRODUCTION

Diet-related chronic diseases account for multiple leading causes of mortality in the United States.[1,2] In their systematic analysis looking at health patterns from 1990 to 2016, the US Burden of Disease Collaborators ranked "dietary risks" as the number one mortality risk factor in 2016.[3] In recent decades, cardiovascular disease (CVD) and cancer have persisted as the 2 leading causes of death, and cerebrovascular

[a] Center for Health Promotion and Disease Prevention, University of North Carolina at Chapel Hill, 1700 Martin Luther King Jr. Boulevard, CB# 7426, Chapel Hill, NC 27599-7426, USA; [b] Department of Nutrition, Gillings School of Global Public Health, University of North Carolina at Chapel Hill, CB# 7461, Chapel Hill, NC, 27599-7461, USA; [c] Division of General Medicine and Clinical Epidemiology, Department of Medicine, School of Medicine, University of North Carolina, CB# 7110, Chapel Hill, NC, 27599-7110, USA
* Corresponding author. Center for Health Promotion and Disease Prevention, University of North Carolina at Chapel Hill, 1700 Martin Luther King Jr. Boulevard, CB# 7426, Chapel Hill, NC 27599-7426.
E-mail address: thomas_keyserling@med.unc.edu

Med Clin N Am 106 (2022) 785–807
https://doi.org/10.1016/j.mcna.2022.05.004
0025-7125/22/© 2022 Elsevier Inc. All rights reserved.

disease and diabetes mellitus have also been major contributors to mortality in the US.[4] Additionally, more than 40% of US adults over 20 years of age have obesity, and a BMI in the obese range increases the risk of developing multiple chronic diseases including type 2 diabetes mellitus, CVD, and some cancers.[5–7]

Primary care providers (PCPs), including advanced care providers, are well-positioned to address the problem of diet-related chronic disease through the continuity of care provided to patients at risk for or diagnosed with chronic diseases. A PCP commonly manages chronic conditions in which the modification of dietary behaviors can have an impact, such as type 2 diabetes mellitus, hypertension, hyperlipidemia, CVD, and obesity.[8] Thus, the ability to assess dietary behaviors of a patient, provide tailored time-efficient dietary counseling, and make appropriate nutrition care referrals are important skills for the PCP. In this article, we will review what constitutes a healthful dietary pattern, how to briefly assess diet during a patient encounter, quick counseling strategies, and when a patient may benefit from a referral to a nutrition specialist. We will also present special considerations when taking a nutrition history.

HEALTHFUL DIETARY PATTERNS

The 2020 to 2025 Dietary Guidelines for Americans emphasize the benefit of healthful dietary patterns for most individuals and the importance of health professionals tailoring dietary recommendations based on individual patient needs.[9] Evidence, mostly from prospective cohort studies, strongly suggests the positive impact of healthful dietary patterns in risk reduction for multiple diet-related chronic diseases, including type 2 diabetes, CVD, some cancers, neurodegenerative disease, and premature mortality.[10] For instance, the Mediterranean-style diet may improve cardiovascular risk factors and outcomes, including blood pressure, lipids, and major cardiovascular events.[11–13] Evidence also links the Mediterranean-style dietary pattern with the prevention of the onset of diabetes and improvements in insulin sensitivity.[12,14] Healthful dietary patterns also have neuroprotective effects, such as improved cognitive function and reduced risk of developing neurodegenerative diseases.[1,15]

Healthful dietary patterns have been characterized by a higher score on diet quality indices including the Healthy Eating Index, Alternative Healthy Eating Index, and the Dietary Approaches to Stop Hypertension (DASH) score, and by patterns evaluated in randomized trials.[10,11,16]

Based on this evidence, a healthful dietary pattern includes:

1. Regular consumption of foods with high-quality fats
2. Regular consumption of foods with high-quality carbohydrates
3. Reduced consumption of poor-quality carbohydrates and processed foods

---

Foods with high-quality fats include nuts, seeds, fish, common inexpensive vegetable oils relatively high in polyunsaturated fats and hereafter termed "common vegetable oils" (eg, canola, soy, corn, and peanut oil), and olive oil. High-quality carbohydrate foods include fruits, nonstarchy vegetables, whole grains, and beans. Foods with poor-quality carbohydrates include sugar-sweetened beverages, refined grains, and many processed foods.

THE ROLE OF THE PRIMARY CARE PROVIDER IN NUTRITION CARE

While the PCP is not a nutrition specialist, practice guidelines endorse the role of the PCP in delivering dietary counseling, referring for more intensive dietary counseling, and supporting team-based nutrition interventions.[17] Patients regard physicians as trusted sources of dietary guidance, and studies demonstrate a positive impact of addressing diet during a primary care visit.[18-24] US Preventive Services Task Force (USPSTF) recommendations reflect the importance of addressing preventive measures such as dietary behaviors. The USPSTF currently recommends "offering or referring adults with CVD risk factors to behavioral counseling interventions to promote a healthy diet and physical activity" (B recommendation).[17] This recommendation specifically applies to adult patients (18 and older) with the following CVD risk factors: hypertension/elevated blood pressure, dyslipidemia, or patients with more than one CVD risk factor, such as in patients with metabolic syndrome.[17] The recommended counseling can be implemented face-to-face by PCPs or physicians can refer patients to specially trained providers such as registered dietitians (RDs).[17] Media- or web-based platforms are also an option for meeting the recommendation.[17] Professional societies, such as the American Heart Association and the American Academy of Family Physicians, also endorse dietary counseling for patients at risk for CVD.[17,25,26] Likewise, the USPSTF recommends that "Clinicians should offer or refer patients with prediabetes to effective prevention interventions."[27] To meet dietary counseling recommendations, nutritional assessment is a critical first step and one that can be achieved during a primary care visit, whether briefly by a clinician or through office supports, which we will review in greater depth.

THE ROLE OF THE REGISTERED DIETITIAN IN NUTRITION CARE

RDs, also known as registered dietitian nutritionists (RDNs), are nutrition specialists highly skilled in nutritional assessment and intervention who provide care in all health care settings.[28] Using nutrition science and medical nutrition therapy (MNT), RDs assist patients by providing in-depth tailored dietary guidance specific to the needs of patients.

The goal of an RD in the primary care setting is to work alongside health care professionals in nutrition-related disease prevention and treatment using the Nutrition Care Process (NCP). The NCP encompasses the following steps: nutrition assessment, nutrition diagnosis, nutrition intervention, and nutrition monitoring and evaluation.[29] Patient-centered interventions an RD might provide include but are not limited to disease-specific nutrition education and counseling, initiation of alternative feeding modalities, and connection to government nutrition programs and community nutrition resources.[29] Patients and physicians benefit not only from the expertise RDs provide in nutrition care but also the amount of time RDs can devote to dietary assessment and counseling, as we will review in greater detail later in discussion.

TEAM-BASED NUTRITION CARE

Interdisciplinary team-based care, such as those using an RD, successfully advances the health of the patient and harnesses the skills and expertise of multiple disciplines in health care.[30-33] Such teams have been shown to improve a patient's access to medical services and nutrition support, patient satisfaction levels, and overall quality of care.[34] In the primary care setting, interprofessional collaboration may alleviate the barrier of time constraints faced by PCPs.

Interdisciplinary nutrition teams usually consist of a PCP, RD, registered nurse, social worker, trained support staff (eg, nurses and care assistants, nutrition and dietetic technicians) and, if appropriate, a mental health provider.[34] PCPs are positioned uniquely in the health care setting as they are often the health care professional with whom patients regularly visit and serve as a gateway for referrals to other health services. This means they are well-suited to both screen and identify patients at nutritional risk, offer focused dietary counseling if time permits, and make appropriate referrals to nutrition specialists. When a referral is indicated, RDs use their expertise in MNT to address the nutritional needs of the patient.[28] Should a patient need to be connected with assistance programs or community nutrition resources such as the Supplemental Nutrition Assistance Program (SNAP) or the Special Supplemental Nutrition Program for Women, Infants, Children (WIC), either an RD, social worker, or medical provider can connect patients. While interdisciplinary teams may look different depending on the resources of a specific health care setting, the goal remains the same: the health of the patient.

Note: If a health care setting lacks an RD, please see the "How to find a registered dietitian" section later in discussion.

NUTRITION ASSESSMENT IN A PRIMARY CARE VISIT

The ability of the PCP to address diet in a primary care visit is often limited by time constraints. Several brief dietary assessment tools have been developed and validated to address this barrier.[35] To decrease time spent administering nutrition assessment tools during the visit, brief screeners can be included as pre-visit questionnaires or can be administered by support staff. Patient responses can guide brief dietary counseling discussions or inform the decision to refer to an RD. Some brief dietary assessment tools also integrate counseling suggestions. When selecting a brief dietary assessment tool, it is important to note validity and reliability, intended patient population, and whether the tool incorporates up-to-date dietary recommendations.

Using a case study as an example, we will review an example of a brief dietary assessment and counseling tool and an approach to dietary counseling that takes into account impact on health outcomes, ease of behavior change, and affordability that were developed by our team of nutrition researchers at the University of North Carolina at Chapel Hill.

Case Example:

Mr. Smith is a 47-year-old male who has come in for his annual visit. He has been your patient for 5 years but many acute health concerns (COVID-19 scares, diverticulitis, and so forth) have prevented you from talking about diet. You note he has a number of diet-related health concerns: type 2 diabetes, hypertension, dyslipidemia, and a family history of heart disease. He is married with 2 teenage children, and his wife is primarily responsible for food shopping and meal preparation. Mr. Smith has a mostly sedentary occupation working a desk job at the post office.

For the past year, he has been taking metformin, an ACE inhibitor, and a statin that you prescribed.

Today, his BMI is 34 and his blood pressure is 138/90 mm Hg (H). His laboratory results from recent bloodwork show:

HbA1C: 6.8% (H)

Total cholesterol: 209 mg/dL (H)

LDL: 166 mg/dL (H)

HDL: 39 md/dL (L)

Triglycerides: 187 mg/dL (H)

During today's visit, the patient does not have acute health concerns, so there is time and context (given his chronic disease profile) to offer brief dietary assessment and counseling.

BRIEF DIETARY ASSESSMENT AND COUNSELING TOOL EXAMPLE

Our research team has developed and adapted the brief diet assessment instrument provided in **Table 1**. We initially called it "Starting the Conversation" and collaborated with others to conduct a validation study in 2011.[36] Given updates in the scientific literature, we adapted this instrument for the Heart Healthy Lenoir Project and subsequently have made some additional modifications.[37] As suggested by its title, this instrument is designed as a quick self-assessment survey (5 minutes) consisting of 10 questions and associated counseling tips, outlined in **Table 1**, that can be used by the provider to initiate a conversation about dietary change. This tool is an example of a brief dietary assessment tool that can be administered as a pre-visit questionnaire or by support staff. It also serves as a nutrition education resource for patients as it provides tips for positive dietary changes. It can be used alone or in conjunction with the Three-Step Framework for Dietary Change described later, depending on the preferences and limitations of providers and health care settings.

THREE-STEP FRAMEWORK FOR DIETARY CHANGE

This brief clinic-based dietary counseling approach prioritizes: (1) specific behavior changes best supported by the literature to reduce the risk for premature mortality and common chronic diseases, (2) dietary changes that are easiest to make and maintain, and (3) affordability. This approach, intended for PCPs, focuses on changes that are impactful, relatively easy to make, and affordable as outlined below in a 3-step sequence for counseling and in **Fig. 1**. The number of steps addressed at any one visit may depend on the patient's stage of change (discussed later in discussion). Here we describe the 3 steps of the dietary framework and a summary of the steps is provided in **Fig. 1**.

Three-Step Framework for Dietary Change:

Step 1–Improve fat quality by increasing the consumption of familiar foods with high-quality fat composition. These changes are easy to make and acceptable to most patients as nuts/nut butters and full-fat salad dressing (major ingredient vegetable oil vs. corn syrup for fat-free alternatives) are highly palatable.[38] Nuts can be expensive, but peanuts, peanut butter, salad dressing, and common vegetable oils are not. Importantly, nuts and seeds are foods associated with large relative risk reductions for coronary heart disease (CHD) while polyunsaturated fat is the type of fat most strongly associated with reduced CHD risk.[11,39] Importantly, there is strong evidence that higher fat diets are not associated with weight gain.[39]

Step 2–Improve carbohydrate quality by choosing familiar foods with high-quality carbohydrates (fruits, vegetables, and whole grains) and healthful alternatives for beverages with poor-quality carbohydrates. Eating familiar fruits and vegetables regularly is a good start. Like nuts and seeds, whole grains comprise another food category for which increased consumption is strongly associated with chronic disease risk reduction, particularly when replacing refined/processed carbohydrates.[40] Eating more whole grains may be challenging for some, but with encouragement most can improve whole-grain intake. Increasing consumption at home can easily be accomplished by purchasing whole-grain products like bread, breakfast cereal, pasta, tortillas, and brown rice when grocery shopping. While reducing sugar-sweetened beverages may be hard for some, a variety of beverage products with less sugar are available. Coffee and tea (unsweetened or lightly sweetened) are acceptable to many and both are associated with risk reduction for chronic diseases.[40]

Step 3– Enhance carbohydrate quality even more by adding beans and additional variety to fruits and vegetables. This step might require new food preparation skills and some of the recommended foods may be too expensive for some to eat on a regular basis. In considering if this step is worth the effort, it is noteworthy that while increased consumption of vegetables, fruits, and beans is associated with decreased risk for common chronic diseases, the strength of this association may be less than for nuts, whole grains, and healthful oils.[40] Of note, roasting familiar and not-so-familiar vegetables in oil, though a new skill for many, is relatively easy to do and is a very useful strategy for increasing vegetable palatability and consumption of high-quality fats.

Step 1 recommendations are easy to achieve, and the evidence is strong that these changes will positively impact health outcomes. Step 2 recommendations are generally straightforward and do not require new food preparation skills. We propose primary care clinicians and/or nurses or medical assistants assess and counsel on these dietary behaviors annually by use of a brief handout, such as the example brief dietary assessment and counseling tool in **Table 1**, or a brief web-based program that includes tailored counseling suggestions. Step 3 recommendations require more nutrition knowledge and educational material in support of behavior change. Knowledgeable and motivated PCPs may want to provide this level of counseling facilitated by easy access to relevant print or web-based materials. However, this step may best be undertaken in collaboration with specially trained staff or RDs.

Case Example: Application of the Brief Dietary Assessment and Counseling Tool and the Three-Step Framework for Dietary Change

While Mr. Smith was in the waiting room, he filled out a brief dietary assessment sheet given to him at check-in. He had the following responses:

1. How many times a WEEK do you eat nuts (like peanuts, almonds, walnuts, or cashews) or nut butters like peanut butter? 0 to 1
2. How many times a DAY do you eat foods that contain vegetable oil (olive, canola, corn, soybean, peanut, and other oils), such as full-fat salad dressing or mayonnaise, food fried or sautéed in vegetable oil, or margarine? 2
3. How many regular sodas, sports drinks, or glasses of sweet tea do you drink each DAY? 1 to 2
4. How often do you eat whole-grain bread, rolls, or tortillas? Rarely
5. How many servings of fruits and vegetables do you eat each DAY? 2 or less
6. How many times a WEEK do you eat fish or beans (like pinto or black beans)? 2 or less
7. What about milk and cheese? Milk at dinner most days, cream cheese on a bagel most mornings
8. What about eggs? Sometimes on the weekends
9. What about fast food? Rarely
10. What about dessert? Only on special occasions

While looking over the responses you highlight some priority areas where you think Mr. Smith could take some steps to improve his diet. You review the responses together and learn that as he has a long commute, he often makes a bagel with cream cheese in the morning that he eats on his way to work with his coffee (with 3 spoonfuls of sugar). At work, he grabs a mid-morning cola and chips from the vending machine because that is what is readily available during his break. To save money, he brings a packed lunch, usually a cold-cut sandwich on white bread with chips or salted pretzels. His wife prepares a usual dinner with meat, starch, and steamed vegetables, but he does not often eat the vegetables because he does not like how they taste. At the end of the day, he likes to relax with a couple of beers and buttered microwave popcorn while watching TV.

Following the Three-Step Framework for Dietary Change, you focus on the first 2 steps at this visit and identify some potential goals Mr. Smith can consider to improve his diet:

Step 1: Improving the quality of dietary fats:
- Replace the cream cheese on his bagel with peanut butter
- Add more nuts to his diet, such as a mid-morning or evening snack
- Add more fish to his diet, such as a tuna sandwich at lunch or fish sautéed in common vegetable oils or olive oil at dinner
- Cook vegetables in common vegetable oils or olive oil
- Try a salad with full-fat salad dressing at dinner

Step 2: Improving the quality of carbohydrates
- Try switching to a whole-grain bagel or whole-grain toast at breakfast and whole-grain bread with sandwiches at lunch
- Reduce the amount of sugar added to his morning coffee (half and half is a better choice)
- Bring fruit to work as a snack or add to packed lunch
- Replace evening snack of buttered microwave popcorn with a small portion of peanuts or mixed nuts

- Replace cola with water
- Replace steamed vegetables with salad (with full-fat salad dressing) at dinner

You also recognized that Mr. Smith might enjoy new preparations of foods, such as roasting vegetables and/or adding a sauce to vegetables to improve the taste. This recommendation may require more time to provide the necessary counseling given the potential new food preparation skills required and may be best covered by an RD.

Before making recommendations, you may want to briefly assess his readiness to change (see *Stages of Change*).

STAGES OF CHANGE

When conducting a nutrition assessment, it can be helpful to note the readiness of the patient to make change, as this may influence adherence to recommendations or referrals.[41] Initiating counseling or referring to an RD when the patient does not recognize an issue is present or believe there is much that can be done about it may not be helpful to the patient or be an efficient use of time for the physician or the RD.

The use of the stages of change from the Transtheoretical Model has the potential to provide positive changes in nutrition assessment and intervention to achieve patient-centered goals.[42,43] **Table 2** illustrates indications from the patient to help the PCP identify the stage of change and potential next steps. Understanding a patient's willingness to change and creating an intervention considering this stage increases the likelihood of patient success. Probably the most important consideration is at the initial "precontemplation" level. If a patient is not convinced a problem exists, dietary counseling or referral may be better addressed at a follow-up visit when the patient is more open to change. The "maintenance" stage is also challenging, so it is worthwhile to briefly check in with patients periodically to offer reinforcement and encouragement even if they seem to be doing well.

Case Example: Stages of Change
  You do a quick assessment of Mr. Smith's stage of change for addressing his diet:
  Physician: "I think there are a few changes you could make that wouldn't be as hard as you might think and would still allow you to enjoy your food. Tell me some thoughts you have about that."
  Mr. Smith: "You know, my daughter's been talking to me about what she's learning in her nutrition class, and I guess I'm ready to try something different."
  Your patient's response reflects the Preparation/Action Stage of Change
  Physician: "That's a great idea. Maybe she can help you with this. Let's talk through a couple of things that you think might be the easiest to change (discuss 1 or 2 goals based on the patient's responses to the previously discussed dietary assessment and counseling tool). I can also set you up to visit with our dietitian who can give you lots of good suggestions."

WHEN TO MAKE A REFERRAL TO A REGISTERED DIETITIAN AND HOW THE REGISTERED DIETITIAN CAN HELP

As previously discussed, a referral to an RD can assist with a lifestyle change when a nutritionally relevant condition is identified, and the patient is contemplating or prepared for change. RDs are trained to use MNT to prevent, treat, and manage a wide variety of conditions.[29,48] MNT may involve directly treating the condition, managing side effects, addressing drug-nutrient interactions, referring to community nutrition programs and more.[29] RDs may also provide other beneficial services including group

Table 1
Brief assessment with counseling tips adapted from the Heart Healthy Lenoir Project[37]

What Do You Usually Eat?	Tips for Healthy Eating
1. How many times a WEEK do you eat nuts (like peanuts, almonds, walnuts, or cashews) or nut butter like peanut butter? □ 3 or more □ 2 □ 0–1	*Choose nuts and nut butters often.* Eat a serving of nuts or nut butter 3 or more times each week. • Peanuts and peanut butter are inexpensive and healthy. • A peanut butter sandwich on whole-wheat bread is a good choice for lunch or snack. • Add nuts to fruit and vegetable dishes or salads. • A serving of nuts is a small handful or 2 tablespoons of nut butter.
2. How many times a DAY do you eat foods that contain vegetable oil (olive, canola, corn, soybean, peanut, and other oils), such as full-fat salad dressing or mayonnaise, food fried or sautéed in vegetable oil, or margarine? □ 3 or more □ 2 □ 0–1	*Eat foods made with vegetable oils daily.* Vegetable oils contain healthy fats. Aim for 2–6 servings per day. • Use regular salad dressing and mayonnaise (which have healthy fats) instead of the low-fat or no-fat options, which contain more sugar. • Fry, sauté, or cook with vegetable oil, including olive, canola, corn, soybean, peanut, or other vegetable oils. Olive oil may have additional health benefits compared with other oils. • Roast vegetables in healthy vegetable oils • If more help is needed to make these changes, consider a referral to an RD
3. How many regular sodas, sports drinks, or glasses of sweet tea do you drink each DAY? □ <1 □ 1–2 □ 3 or more	*Choose drinks with less sugar.* Sweet tea, sports drinks, regular sodas, and most fancy coffee drinks contain a lot of sugar (9 teaspoons per 12 ounces of soda). • Water is always a good choice. • Coffee and tea are good choices. A little milk or half and half in coffee or tea is fine, but limit sugar to no more than 2–3 teaspoons per cup or glass. Half unsweetened and half-sweetened tea is a good option. • 100% fruit juice is another good choice, but limit to 1 glass (8 oz) a day.
4. How often do you eat whole-grain bread, rolls, or tortillas? □ Usually □ Sometimes □ Rarely	Choose whole-grain products often. • Eat whole-grain bread instead of white bread whenever possible. • Eat other whole-grain products like whole-wheat pasta, whole-grain tortillas, whole-grain breakfast cereal, and brown rice.
5. How many servings of fruits and vegetables do you eat each DAY? □ 5 or more □ 3–4 □ 2 or less	Eat fruit and vegetables often. • Aim for 5 or more servings of fruits and vegetables each day. • Eat a variety of fruits and vegetables. Try to eat a "rainbow" of colors, including dark green and orange vegetables. • Eat fruit instead of drinking fruit juice.

(continued on next page)

Table 1
(continued)

What Do You Usually Eat?	Tips for Healthy Eating
	• If more help is needed to make these changes, consider a referral to an RD

6. How many times a WEEK do you eat fish or beans (like pinto or black beans)?
    ☐ 5 or more
    ☐ 3–4
    ☐ 2 or less
	Eat fish and beans often and limit intake of red and processed meats.
	• Try to eat fish (including tuna) at least once a week[a].
	• Use vegetable oil to fry fish.
	• One serving a day of red meat or pork is fine.
	• Limit processed meats like bacon, sausage, cold cuts (deli meats), and hot dogs to twice a week.

7. What about milk and cheese?	Consume low- *or* full-fat milk or dairy products such as yogurt or cheese. • You may have heard that no-fat or low-fat dairy products are the best choices, but recent research suggests full-fat dairy products do not increase the risk for heart disease. • Due to high sugar content, limit dairy desserts to a couple of times a week. • Butter is OK, but margarine made with vegetable oil is a slightly better choice.
8. What about eggs?	Eating 1–2 eggs a day is fine. • You may have heard that eating eggs can raise your cholesterol, but recent research suggests eating eggs does not increase the risk for heart disease.
9. What about fast food?	Make healthy choices when dining out. • Limit sugar-sweetened beverages, as noted above. • Enjoy a burger or sandwich as your meal, on a whole-wheat bun or bread, if available. Pizza with veggies is a reasonable choice, as are most entrées at sit-down restaurants. • Consider a side other than fries or potatoes, such as salad, fruit, or vegetables. • If you order fries or dessert, get a small portion or share a larger one.
10. What about dessert?	Make good dessert choices. • Fruit is a good choice for dessert. • Chocolate may reduce the risk of heart disease and dark chocolate may do so more than regular chocolate. Small amounts of dark chocolate (more than 50% cocoa solids), such as half to one ounce, is a good choice for dessert. • Limit cakes and cookies and dairy desserts like ice cream and frozen yogurt to a couple of times a week.

(continued on next page)

Table 1
(continued)

What Do You Usually Eat?	Tips for Healthy Eating
	• Be aware of portion sizes. Consider sharing desserts.

[a] If pregnant or planning a pregnancy, do not eat fish with high mercury content, such as king mackerel, swordfish, and albacore tuna.

	Focus	Sample Behavior Change	Barriers	Sample Counseling Tips
STEP 1	Improve fat quality by increasing the consumption of familiar foods with high-quality fat composition. Impact Ease Affordabiliy[a]	Eat peanuts, tree nuts, and/or nut butters at least 3 times a week.	• Knowledge	• Peanuts and peanut butter are inexpensive and healthful. • Add nuts to fruit and vegetable dishes or salads.
		Eat foods with healthful fats (like avocados and fish) or made with vegetable oils. Aim for 2–6 servings a day.	• Knowledge • Misconception that high-fat foods are not healthful	• Sauté, fry, or cook with olive or common vegetable oils and use margarine made with these oils. • Replace fat-free dressings and spreads with "regular" versions which are made with vegetable oils. • Extra virgin olive oil may have additional health benefits compared with other vegetable oils.
STEP 2	Improve carbohydrate quality by choosing familiar foods with high-quality carbs (fruits, vegetables, and whole grains) and alternatives for beverages with poor quality carbs. Impact Ease Affordability	Eat familiar fruits and vegetables daily. Aim for 5 or more servings each day.	• Perceived palatability and cost	• Eat fruit instead of drinking fruit juice. • Eat larger servings of favorite vegetables to replace poor quality foods. • Frozen vegetables are often an inexpensive option.
		Replace white bread with whole-wheat bread and choose whole grains more often.	• Knowledge • Acceptance of different taste and textures • Different cooking characteristics	• Eat whole-grain bread instead of white bread whenever possible. • Increase the consumption of other whole-grain products including whole-grain pasta, tortillas, breakfast cereals and brown rice.
		Choose drinks with less sugar.	• "Kicking the habit" • Acceptance of healthful alternatives	• Water is always a good choice. • Coffee and tea are good choices. A little milk or cream is fine but limit sugar to 1–2 teaspoons per cup.
STEP 3	Enhance carbohydrate quality even more by adding beans and additional variety to fruits and vegetables. Impact Ease Affordability	Eat beans 3 times a week. Choose dark green and nonstarchy vegetables. Add different types of fruits to what you usually eat.	• Knowledge • Acceptance of different products • Food prep skills • Concern about flatus • "Shelf-life" • Cost	• Try pinto, black, kidney or other beans. Canned beans require less prep time. • Try collard, mustard, or turnip greens. • Make salads with dark green leafy vegetables including lettuce, spinach and/or kale. • Choose fruits like berries, melons, peaches, pears, and plums. • Try roasting vegetables using olive and other oils—this enhances their taste and adds high-quality fats to the diet.

Fig. 1. Three-step framework for dietary change emphasizing impact on health outcomes, ease of behavior change, and affordability. Graphic qualitatively conveys (from *left to right*) greater health impact, ease of making dietary behavior changes (familiarity with food and preparation time or skill), and affordability. [a]Though extra virgin olive oil and tree nuts can be expensive, peanuts, peanut butter, common vegetable oils (canola, soybean, corn, and peanut) and familiar products made with common vegetable oils (eg, full-fat salad dressing and mayonnaise) are inexpensive.

Table 2
Nutrition stages of change and recommendations[44-47]

	Definition	Potential Signs	Tips for Brief Encounter	Example Scenario
Precontemplation	Unaware of or in denial about the harmfulness of behavior with no intention to change	• Does not believe harm applies to self • Denial of the magnitude of consequences • Feels unable to control condition • Arms crossed, slouching, aggression or reservation	• Encourage reevaluation of current beliefs • Schedule patient for a return visit to reassess readiness	Patient: "I don't think my high blood sugar is something to worry about." Physician: "Tell me a bit about why you think it's nothing to worry about."
Contemplation	Aware of behavior and its consequences, thinking about change, no action taken to change	• Considers change but states reasons not to change • No effort to make changes despite recognition	• Note discrepancies between goals and choices • Explore both positive and negative aspects of making change • Begin to explore what change might look like • Schedule patient for a return visit to reassess readiness • Suggest referral to RD	Patient: "I know my high blood sugar is an issue, but I really enjoy sweets. I don't want to give them up." Physician: "It's true, change can be hard. I think we can find alternatives you would enjoy without completely giving up sweets."
Preparation	Intends to make changes in the next month	• States willingness to make change • Acknowledges positives of change outweigh negatives • Develops plan to change	• Note commitment to change • Have patient identify potential ways to change before offering a range of change ideas • Encourage small first steps in setting goals • Note barriers and supports to change • Referral to RD	Patient: "I think I'm ready to fix my blood sugar. I'm tired of dealing with it and I don't want it to impact my life anymore." Physician: "I'm happy to hear this. Let's talk about some ways you could take the first step in blood sugar management."

(continued on next page)

Table 2
(continued)

	Definition	Potential Signs	Tips for Brief Encounter	Example Scenario
Action	Making impactful changes in behavior	• Actively making changes to address condition or goals	• Review progress on goals • Identify potential barriers that may arise and coping strategies • Identify support systems and how they might be used • Inquire about progress	Patient: "Since I last saw you. I've increased the amount of fiber in my diet and reduced my intake of soda." Physician: "That's great news! Tell me more about how it's going."
Maintenance	Behavior change sustained for at least 6 months	• Maintaining changes and progress • Actively using support systems • Potentially using multiple strategies to maintain change	• Continue to offer support • Inquire about progress • Identify potential barriers that may lead to relapse • Actively assist in growing skills	Patient: "I've been doing well on my blood sugar goals. I go to a potluck on Wednesdays and started bringing an Italian pasta salad with less noodles and more veggies and beans. Everyone really likes it." Physician: "That's a great strategy Keep me posted on how this goes."

cooking and nutrition classes and nutrition support groups to help multiple patients manage their conditions.

Once instance when MNT is indicated is when required nutrition changes are outside the scope of what the PCP can address during routine visits, as outlined in Step 3 of the Three-Step Framework for Dietary Change above. Dietary counseling addressing unfamiliar foods or new food preparation skills is best conducted by an RD as well as counseling for complex conditions that require knowledge of MNT. For example, consistent use of MNT has been shown to significantly improve markers of dyslipidemia, management of diabetes, and gastrointestinal conditions, and is a cost-effective means to do so.[49-51] A physician may also consider a referral to compliment medication or when a patient wishes not to use medication.

HOW TO FIND A REGISTERED DIETITIAN

RDs may be readily accessible as staff members of a primary care clinic, the clinic's health care system network, local health departments, or local health clubs or may work in private practice. The Academy of Nutrition and Dietetics provides a "Find a Nutrition Expert" resource to help find nutrition experts by location, insurance coverage, specialty, and language needs.

> For help identifying a nutrition expert, visit the "Find a Nutrition Expert" resource here: https://www.eatright.org/find-a-nutrition-expert

---

Case Example: RD referral

Mr. Smith's wife and daughter join him for his first visit with the dietitian as they are all interested in making healthier food choices and his wife prepares most of his meals.

Dietitian: "It's great to hear that not only are you interested in making a change, Mr. Smith, but that you have the support of your family as well. Share with me a bit about what's going on and what you'd like to get out of the appointment with me today."

Mr. Smith: "The doc suggested that now might be a good time to work on my diet now that I have some other areas of my health under control. I have diabetes and high blood pressure, and heart disease runs in my family. I'm a bit nervous about this and I don't want to give up foods that I enjoy."

Dietitian: "You should be proud of yourself for taking this initiative. Let's try to make some changes that are acceptable to you and your family. Here is the dietary assessment you filled out at your primary care physician's office with some areas highlighted that we could work on. Tell me what you're the most comfortable addressing."

Mr. Smith: "Well I really don't like vegetables and I'm iffy on fruits, but I think I'd be open to trying whole-grain breads. Maybe I can start by doing that at lunch with my sandwich. Honey, do you think we can buy whole-grain bread?"

Mrs Smith: "I think we can try it out. Maybe I can use it for my toast in the morning."

Dietitian: "I think that is a great idea. Foods with whole grains can help improve blood sugar, reduce the risk of heart disease, and prevent diverticulosis from worsening. Let's set a goal around this, and in the future, I can show you some ways to make fruits and vegetables tasty. I'll see you in 2 weeks."

The dietitian reports back to you the changes and progress on Mr. Smith's dietary habits.

Physician: "Mr. Smith, your laboratories are improving."

Mr. Smith: "I feel better doc. I'd actually like to talk to you about reducing my Metformin dosage. Is that something you think I can do eventually?"

Physician: "I don't see why not with the track you are on. Let's keep at this progress and see where you're at next visit."

NUTRITION CARE ACCESS

An important consideration with an RD referral is access to and reimbursement for care. Depending on a patient's insurance, age, and disease condition, insurance may or may not cover MNT treatment.[52] See **Box 1** for more information about RD visit coverage by insurance types.

Of note, through the Intensive Behavioral Therapy program,[54,55] Medicare also covers the delivery of behavioral counseling for obesity in face-to-face visits by PCPs with the following frequency:

- Month 1: weekly visits
- Months 2 to 6: visits every other week

Medicare recipients eligible for this benefit may continue with monthly visits for months 7 to 12 if they meet the weight loss requirement.[54,55]

> For more information about state-specific nutrition care regulations please visit:
> https://www.eatrightpro.org/about-us/what-is-an-rdn-and-dtr/work-with-an-rdn-or-dtr/referring-patients-to-an-rdn

SPECIAL CONSIDERATIONS
Eating Disorders

Given PCPs may see patients more regularly than many other health care providers, they are well-positioned to identify patients with eating disorders (EDs) and disordered eating. Individuals with disordered eating may show many of the same signs and symptoms as clinical EDs, but in a less severe form. For example, an individual may binge eat once a week for 2 months and purge every other week, which would not meet the DSM-V criteria for a diagnosable bulimia nervosa, yet the individual still has a significant mental health concern.

Individuals are often skilled at hiding their symptoms or withholding information, as EDs often serve a purpose for an individual whether it is control, physical (eg, a

---

Box 1
Information about RD insurance coverage

Medicare[52]
- Covers outpatient MNT for beneficiaries with diabetes, chronic renal insufficiency/end-stage renal disease (nondialysis renal disease), or post kidney transplant.
- Patient must have a physician order to receive coverage from an RD.
- Referral should include diagnosis and disease codes, recent laboratory data and medications, referral form, and documented need for MNT in the patient's medical chart.
- Medicare only allows 3 hours of MNT in the first year and 2 hours in the years following.
- Repeat previous steps to obtain more hours.

Medicaid[53]
- Affordable Care Act covers MNT under the "Preventive and Wellness Services" category for dietary counseling for adults at risk for chronic disease and obesity screening and counseling for all age groups.
- Coverage varies by state and specific Medicaid plans.

Private Insurance[52]
- Different private insurances and states possess different criteria for MNT reimbursement.
- Referral may be required.
- Check with the specific private insurer and state in which care is delivered to confirm what is needed.

Table 3
Common signs and symptoms of eating disorders in males and females[60–63]

Emotional and Behavioral:
- A desire/effort to lose weight or diet
- Preoccupation with weight, body shape and size, and food
- Meal skipping or delayed eating
- Social withdrawal
- Excessive exercise
- Stress over gender identity
- Use of laxatives or diuretics
- Excessive use of water, calorie-free drinks, and gum
- Excessive caffeine or hot beverage intake
- Skipping insulin doses

Physical:
- Visible weight changes
- Gastrointestinal issues
- Irregular or absent menstrual cycle
- Abnormal electrolytes, liver enzymes, hematological markers, blood glucose, cholesterol levels, blood arterial gases, testosterone levels, thyroid studies, or vitamin D levels
- Scarred fingers and/or enamel erosion
- Dry and brittle skin, hair, and nails
- Small, fine hairs (lanugo)
- Growth retardation
- Osteoporosis and/or fractures
- Enlarged salivary glands

desirable appearance), biological (eg, lack of menstrual cycle), or other outcomes. Recognizing the signs and symptoms in **Table 3** requires a health care professional to critically consider presenting factors. Warning signs may warrant speaking with family members in a HIPPA-compliant manner to understand if other signs and symptoms are occurring.

EDs can occur in any gender or ethnicity and at any age. Emerging research shows that EDs may be as common or potentially more common in minorities.[56,57] In many non-White cultures, mental health and mental health conditions are not spoken about in the home, so providers may consider speaking with the patient alone if family or significant others are present.[58] Males are also susceptible to EDs.[59]

As it may be challenging to diagnose EDs, we suggest using validated screening instruments. Here we will introduce brief screening questionnaires that can be easily integrated into a primary care visit. An important consideration is that most tools were developed with White women, which could lead to missing positive cases in other genders and races/ethnicities. In the appropriate context, if a patient exhibits signs or symptoms suggestive of an ED (see **Table 3**), a physician may consider using a brief screening questionnaire such as those listed in **Box 2**.

If a patient screens positive for an ED, the PCP should make referrals to appropriate health professionals with expertise in the management of EDs. It is likely that this team

Box 2
Common eating disorder screening questionnaires in primary care

- Sick, Control, One, Fat, Food (SCOFF)[64]
  - Five-item freely accessible screening tool for the general population
  - Published in multiple languages
- Eating Disorder Examination Questionnaire (EDE-Q)[65,66]
  - 28-item freely accessible screening tool suitable for those over 14 years of age
  - Published in multiple languages
- Eating Disorder Examination Questionnaire Short (EDE-QS)[67]
  - 12-item freely accessible screening tool for the general population
  - Published in multiple languages

will include a mental health specialist (eg, psychologist, psychiatrist, social worker, licensed therapist), an RD (eg, certified eating disorder registered dietitian [CEDRD]), and MD, PA, or NP specializing in ED treatment. If no mental health specialists with appropriate expertise are known, a provider may use findedhelp.com.

Weight Stigma

As the number of individuals with overweight and obesity rises, it is important to consider the potential for weight stigma in the health care setting. Weight stigma is defined as internalized or actualized demeaning, discriminatory beliefs or behaviors toward individuals in larger bodies.[68] In the health care setting, this may manifest as the notion that individuals in larger bodies are lazy or lack self-control.[69] At times the health care setting itself can cause an individual to feel stigmatized. This includes an environment with unaccommodating seating, gowns, and blood pressure cuffs.

It is important to be cognizant of weight bias which may lead to poor health care utilization, provider mistrust, disordered eating, alcohol use, weight gain, and other negative health outcomes.[70] One can circumvent the potential for weight stigma by becoming aware of and managing one's biases toward those in larger bodies, using respectful, person-first language (eg, individual in a larger body rather than obese individual), participating in a training on weight stigma, asking the patient for permission to talk about their weight, and creating a medical environment that is welcoming to those in larger bodies.[71] The UConn RUDD Center for Food, Policy, and Health offers trainings, presentations, handouts, and other resources for health care professionals on managing weight bias in health care.[72]

Food Insecurity

Given increasing concern about food insecurity, many clinical settings are now using the two-item screener—the Hunger Vital Sign Survey—to screen patients, and the questions are included in some of the major electronic medical record systems such as EPIC.[73] However, the questions are rarely asked. Providers can increase focus on this by creating systems to make sure the questions are asked and responses recorded. When identifying options for nutrition referrals, it is also helpful to identify sources of information for local resources such as food pantries and federal nutrition programs to address food insecurity. Food banks and pantries are making significant improvements in the nutritional quality of the food made available.[74]

Hunger Vital Sign Survey[73]
  2-item screener for food insecurity
  1. Within the past 12 months, we worried whether our food would run out before we got money to buy more
     ☐ often true ☐ sometimes true ☐ never true ☐ don't know/refused
  2. Within the past 12 months, the food we bought just didn't last and we didn't have money to get more.
     ☐ often true ☐ sometimes true ☐ never true ☐ don't know/refused

---

Supplements

Dietary supplements are beneficial for a limited number of medical conditions; however, data from the 2017 to 2018 National Health and Nutrition Examination Survey show 57.6% of adults 20 years and older in the United States used a dietary supplement in the last 30 days.[75] This prevalence increases with age and may be higher in women such that 80.2% of women aged 60 and older had used a dietary supplement in the last 30 days.[75] Dietary supplements can have unintended consequences when taken without proper consideration. For example, some vitamin and mineral supplements often contain concentrations well beyond the Dietary Reference Intakes (DRIs) set by the Food and Nutrition Board, potentially placing individuals at risk for toxicities. Despite the Food and Drug Administration (FDA) having the purview to test products once they are on the market, they do not test products before market entry nor do they test every product sold to consumers.[76] This places consumers at risk for using potentially harmful products. Thus, it is advised that physicians also inquire about dietary supplements when asking a patient about medication usage. Many RDs are well-versed in dietary supplements and may be a beneficial resource when identifying if a dietary supplement is right for a patient.

For more information on specific dietary supplements:
- Visit the National Institute of Health Office of Dietary Supplements' Dietary Supplement Label Database: https://dsld.od.nih.gov/
- View the Walt Larimore MD, Dónal O'Mathúna's article, "Dietary Supplements – The Wild West of Good, Bad, and a Whole Lotta Ugly," in this series

---

INNOVATIVE MODELS FOR NUTRITION CARE

To address the need for increased access to and utilization of nutrition care as well as specific needs of patients, several innovative models of nutrition care delivery have been developed. Some examples of innovative nutrition care models are outlined in **Box 3**.

NUTRITION TRAINING OPPORTUNITIES FOR PHYSICIANS

Several nutrition training opportunities are available to physicians, including short on-line courses,[83] conferences,[84,85] and board certification as a Physician Nutrition Specialist.[86] Many opportunities offer continuing medical education (CME) credit. A growing number of medical training programs are introducing or increasing nutrition education opportunities at the undergraduate, graduate, and continuing medical education levels with a focus on training in dietary behavior assessment and change, often in the context of "Food as Medicine" or "Culinary Medicine."[87]

Box 3
Examples of innovative models for nutrition care

Shared medical appointments:
Patients with shared diagnoses receive medical care in a group setting for a longer visit, allowing for more time to devote to nutrition education. These group visits can be co-led by physicians and RDs and can include cooking demonstrations.[77]

Nutrition education and cooking classes:
Providers may refer patients to community cooking classes with integrated nutrition education. Classes may also be delivered by trained health professionals and can be offered virtually.[78]

Healthy food prescription programs:
In general, providers prescribe healthy food, usually fresh produce, and administer vouchers that patients can redeem at farmers' markets and/or grocery stores.[79]

Medically tailored meal programs:
Generally intended for patients with complex medical needs and limitations securing meals, medically tailored meal programs regularly deliver meals tailored to the specific health needs of a patient, with benefits of diet quality improvement, reduced food insecurity, and lower health care expenditures.[80–82]

SUMMARY

Poor diet quality is a contributing factor to several of the leading causes of morbidity and mortality in the US, and PCPs frequently manage conditions in which dietary change can make an impact. Dietary assessment is a critical skill for PCPs to identify patients in need of additional nutrition care. PCPs can achieve nutrition assessment through brief dietary assessment tools, some of which integrate brief counseling tips such as the example reviewed in this article. Counseling can be brief and prioritized by the impact of the dietary change on health outcomes, the ease of the behavior change, and affordability. To increase efficiency, providers can rely on office supports to integrate dietary assessment when time is a limiting factor. Team-based approaches can improve the overall quality of nutrition care patients receive. In particular, RDs are nutrition specialists and valuable resources for patients and providers. PCPs also have an important role in the management of other nutrition-related concerns such as eating disorders, food insecurity, and supplement use. These conditions are identified by taking an appropriate history or using reliable screening instruments. Once identified, referral to another health professional such as an RD may be appropriate.

CLINICS CARE POINTS

- Following a healthful dietary pattern can positively impact chronic disease risk, particularly for type 2 diabetes, cardiovascular disease, and some cancers.
- The US Preventive Services Task Force recommendations regarding cardiovascular disease risk and prediabetes screening highlight the benefits of behavioral counseling and preventive interventions.
- Multiple brief dietary assessment tools have been developed and validated to address time constraints of patient visits; however, whether the tools reflect up-to-date recommendations needs to be considered.
- Screening for diet quality, particularly focusing on the quality of fats and carbohydrates, can identify impactful, easy, and affordable potential goals patients can set toward healthful dietary change.
- Nutrition screening in a primary care visit can help identify patients who would benefit from a referral to an RD for more comprehensive nutritional assessment and treatment, including medical nutrition therapy.
- RDs can provide counseling that improves the management of diet-related health conditions, especially those that may require highly tailored counseling such as diabetes, gastrointestinal conditions, and dyslipidemia.
- Several validated tools for eating disorder screening are available to help identify patients in need of referral to specialized care.
- Screening for food insecurity and supplement usage may reveal information important to the medical care of the patient.

ACKNOWLEDGMENTS

Research informing the content of the article was done with support from National Institutes of Health (NIH) grant 5P50 HL105184 to the University of North Carolina Center for Health Promotion and Disease Prevention (HPDP). Other support was provided by Centers for Disease Control and Prevention (CDC) cooperative agreement No. U48/DP001944 to HPDP (a CDC Prevention Research Center).

DISCLOSURE

The authors have nothing to disclose.

REFERENCES

1. Morze J, Danielewicz A, Hoffmann G, et al. Diet quality as assessed by the healthy eating index, alternate healthy eating index, dietary approaches to stop hypertension score, and health outcomes: a second update of a systematic review and meta-analysis of cohort studies. J Acad Nutr Diet 2020;120(12): 1998–2031.e15.
2. About Chronic Diseases | CDC. Available at: https://www.cdc.gov/ chronicdisease/about/index.htm. Accessed April 5, 2022.
3. US Burden of Disease Collaborators, Mokdad AH, Ballestros K, et al. The State of US Health, 1990-2016: Burden of Diseases, Injuries, and Risk Factors Among US States. JAMA 2018;319(14):1444–72.
4. Table 6, Leading causes of death and numbers of deaths, by sex, race, and Hispanic origin: United States, 1980 and 2018 - Health, United States, 2019 - NCBI Bookshelf. Available at: https://www.ncbi.nlm.nih.gov/books/NBK569311/table/ ch3.tab6/?report=objectonly. Accessed March 7, 2022.
5. Hales CM, Carroll MD, Fryar CD, et al. Prevalence of Obesity and Severe Obesity Among Adults: United States, 2017-2018. NCHS Data Brief 2020;(360):1–8.
6. Obesity and Cancer | CDC. Available at: https://www.cdc.gov/cancer/obesity/ index.htm. Accessed March 7, 2022.
7. Powell-Wiley TM, Poirier P, Burke LE, et al. Obesity and cardiovascular disease: A scientific statement from the american heart association. Circulation 2021; 143(21):e984–1010.
8. Santo L, Okeyode T. National Ambulatory Medical Care Survey: 2018 National Summary Tables. Available at: https://www.cdc.gov/nchs/data/ahcd/namcs_ summary/2018-namcs-web-tables-508.pdf.
9. U.S. Department of Agriculture and U.S. Department of Health and Human Services. Dietary guidelines for Americans, 2020-2025. 9th edition. U.S. Department of Agriculture and U.S. Department of Health and Human Services; 2020. Available at: DietaryGuidelines.gov.
10. Schwingshackl L, Bogensberger B, Hoffmann G. Diet Quality as Assessed by the Healthy Eating Index, Alternate Healthy Eating Index, Dietary Approaches to Stop Hypertension Score, and Health Outcomes: An Updated Systematic Review and Meta-Analysis of Cohort Studies. J Acad Nutr Diet 2018;118(1):74–100.e11.
11. Estruch R, Ros E, Salas-Salvadó J, et al. Primary Prevention of Cardiovascular Disease with a Mediterranean Diet Supplemented with Extra-Virgin Olive Oil or Nuts. N Engl J Med 2018;378(25):e34.
12. Ros E, Martínez-González MA, Estruch R, et al. Mediterranean diet and cardiovascular health: Teachings of the PREDIMED study. Adv Nutr 2014;5(3):330S–6S.
13. Kesse-Guyot E, Ahluwalia N, Lassale C, et al. Adherence to Mediterranean diet reduces the risk of metabolic syndrome: a 6-year prospective study. Nutr Metab Cardiovasc Dis 2013;23(7):677–83.
14. Martínez-González MA, Salas-Salvadó J, Estruch R, et al. Benefits of the mediterranean diet: insights from the PREDIMED study. Prog Cardiovasc Dis 2015;58(1): 50–60.
15. Valls-Pedret C, Sala-Vila A, Serra-Mir M, et al. Mediterranean Diet and Age-Related Cognitive Decline: A Randomized Clinical Trial. JAMA Intern Med 2015;175(7):1094–103.

16. de Lorgeril M, Renaud S, Mamelle N, et al. Mediterranean alpha-linolenic acid-rich diet in secondary prevention of coronary heart disease. Lancet 1994; 343(8911):1454–9.

17. US Preventive Services Task Force, Krist AH, Davidson KW, et al. Behavioral counseling interventions to promote a healthy diet and physical activity for cardiovascular disease prevention in adults with cardiovascular risk factors: US preventive services task force recommendation statement. JAMA 2020;324(20): 2069–75.

18. Delichatsios HK, Hunt MK, Lobb R, et al. EatSmart: efficacy of a multifaceted preventive nutrition intervention in clinical practice. Prev Med 2001;33(2 Pt 1):91–8.

19. Hunt MK, Lobb R, Delichatsios HK, et al. Process evaluation of a clinical preventive nutrition intervention. Prev Med 2001;33(2 Pt 1):82–90.

20. Ockene IS, Hebert JR, Ockene JK, et al. Effect of physician-delivered nutrition counseling training and an office-support program on saturated fat intake, weight, and serum lipid measurements in a hyperlipidemic population: Worcester Area Trial for Counseling in Hyperlipidemia (WATCH). Arch Intern Med 1999; 159(7):725–31.

21. Beresford SA, Curry SJ, Kristal AR, et al. A dietary intervention in primary care practice: the Eating Patterns Study. Am J Public Health 1997;87(4):610–6.

22. International Food Information Council Foundation. 2018 Food & Health Survey.; 2018.

23. Kreuter MW, Chheda SG, Bull FC. How does physician advice influence patient behavior? Evidence for a priming effect. Arch Fam Med 2000;9(5):426–33.

24. Huang J, Yu H, Marin E, et al. Physicians' weight loss counseling in two public hospital primary care clinics. Acad Med 2004;79(2):156–61.

25. Arnett DK, Blumenthal RS, Albert MA, et al. 2019 ACC/AHA guideline on the primary prevention of cardiovascular disease: A report of the american college of cardiology/american heart association task force on clinical practice guidelines. Circulation 2019;140(11):e596–646.

26. Healthful Diet and Physical Activity to Prevent Cardiovascular Disease (CVD). Available at: https://www.aafp.org/family-physician/patient-care/clinical-recommendations/all-clinical-recommendations/diet-cvd.html. Accessed January 17, 2022.

27. US Preventive Services Task Force, Davidson KW, Barry MJ, et al. Screening for prediabetes and type 2 diabetes: US preventive services task force recommendation statement. JAMA 2021;326(8):736–43.

28. Academy Quality Management Committee. Academy of nutrition and dietetics: revised 2017 scope of practice for the registered dietitian nutritionist. J Acad Nutr Diet 2018;118(1):141–65.

29. Academy of Nutrition and Dietetics. Nutrition Terminology Reference Manual (eNCPT): Dietetics Language for Nutrition Care. Available at: http://ncpt.webauthor.com. Accessed March 21, 2022.

30. Hoekstra JC, Goosen JHM, de Wolf GS, et al. Effectiveness of multidisciplinary nutritional care on nutritional intake, nutritional status and quality of life in patients with hip fractures: a controlled prospective cohort study. Clin Nutr 2011;30(4): 455–61.

31. Lee JS, Kang JE, Park SH, et al. Nutrition and clinical outcomes of nutrition support in multidisciplinary team for critically ill patients. Nutr Clin Pract 2018;33(5): 633–9.

32. Sneve J, Kattelmann K, Ren C, et al. Implementation of a multidisciplinary team that includes a registered dietitian in a neonatal intensive care unit improved nutrition outcomes. Nutr Clin Pract 2008;23(6):630–4.

33. Martin OJ, Wu W-C, Taveira TH, et al. Multidisciplinary group behavioral and pharmacologic intervention for cardiac risk reduction in diabetes: a pilot study. Diabetes Educ 2007;33(1):118–27.

34. Yinusa G, Scammell J, Murphy J, et al. Multidisciplinary Provision of Food and Nutritional Care to Hospitalized Adult In-Patients: A Scoping Review. J Multidiscip Healthc 2021;14:459–91.

35. England CY, Andrews RC, Jago R, et al. A systematic review of brief dietary questionnaires suitable for clinical use in the prevention and management of obesity, cardiovascular disease and type 2 diabetes. Eur J Clin Nutr 2015;69(9): 977–1003.

36. Paxton AE, Strycker LA, Toobert DJ, et al. Starting the conversation performance of a brief dietary assessment and intervention tool for health professionals. Am J Prev Med 2011;40(1):67–71.

37. Thayer LM, Pimentel DC, Smith JC, et al. Eating Well While Dining Out: Collaborating with Local Restaurants to Promote Heart Healthy Menu Items. Am J Health Educ 2017;48(1):11–21.

38. Keyserling TC, Samuel-Hodge CD, Pitts SJ, et al. A community-based lifestyle and weight loss intervention promoting a Mediterranean-style diet pattern evaluated in the stroke belt of North Carolina: the Heart Healthy Lenoir Project. BMC Public Health 2016;16:732.

39. Estruch R, Ros E. The role of the Mediterranean diet on weight loss and obesity-related diseases. Rev Endocr Metab Disord 2020;21(3):315–27.

40. Mozaffarian D. Dietary and policy priorities for cardiovascular disease, diabetes, and obesity: A comprehensive review. Circulation 2016;133(2):187–225.

41. Mochari-Greenberger H, Terry MB, Mosca L. Does stage of change modify the effectiveness of an educational intervention to improve diet among family members of hospitalized cardiovascular disease patients? J Am Diet Assoc 2010; 110(7):1027–35.

42. Nakabayashi J, Melo GR-I, Toral N. Transtheoretical model-based nutritional interventions in adolescents: a systematic review. BMC Public Health 2020;20(1): 1543.

43. Carvalho de Menezes M, Bedeschi LB, Santos LCD, et al. Interventions directed at eating habits and physical activity using the Transtheoretical Model: a systematic review. Nutr Hosp 2016;33(5):586.

44. Prochaska JO, DiClemente CC, Norcross JC. In search of how people change. Applications to addictive behaviors. Am Psychol 1992;47(9):1102–14.

45. Miller WR, Rollnick S. Motivational interviewing: preparing people to change addictive behavior. 1st edition. New York: The Guilford Press; 1991. p. 348.

46. Zimmerman GL, Olsen CG, Bosworth MF. A "stages of change" approach to helping patients change behavior. Am Fam Physician 2000;61(5):1409–16.

47. The Transtheoretical Model (Stages of Change). Available at: https://sphweb. bumc.bu.edu/otlt/mph-modules/sb/behavioralchangetheories/ behavioralchangetheories6.html. Accessed March 8, 2022.

48. Definition of Terms Task Force, Quality Management Committee Board of Directors. Academy of Nutrition and Dietetics Definition of Terms List. February 2021.

49. Franz MJ, Powers MA, Leontos C, et al. The evidence for medical nutrition therapy for type 1 and type 2 diabetes in adults. J Am Diet Assoc 2010;110(12): 1852–89.

50. Sikand G, Cole RE, Handu D, et al. Clinical and cost benefits of medical nutrition therapy by registered dietitian nutritionists for management of dyslipidemia: A systematic review and meta-analysis. J Clin Lipidol 2018;12(5):1113–22.
51. Academy of Nutrition and Dietetics. Medical Nutrition Therapy Effectiveness Systematic Review (2013-2015). Evidence Analysis Library. 2015. Available at: https://www.andeal.org/topic.cfm?menu=5284&cat=3808. Accessed January 23, 2022.
52. Referring Patients to an RDN. Available at: https://www.eatrightpro.org/about-us/what-is-an-rdn-and-dtr/work-with-an-rdn-or-dtr/referring-patients-to-an-rdn. Accessed March 7, 2022.
53. Medicaid and RDNs. Available at: https://www.eatrightpro.org/payment/nutrition-services/medicaid/medicaid-and-rdns#1. Accessed March 7, 2022.
54. The National Council on Aging. Available at: https://www.ncoa.org/article/obesity-treatment-and-medicare-a-guide-to-understanding-coverage. Accessed March 7, 2022.
55. Improve the chances of your Medicare claims for obesity counseling. Available at: https://www.aafp.org/journals/fpm/blogs/gettingpaid/entry/improve_the_chances_your_medicare.html. Accessed March 7, 2022.
56. Goode RW, Cowell MM, Mazzeo SE, et al. Binge eating and binge-eating disorder in Black women: A systematic review. Int J Eat Disord 2020;53(4):491–507.
57. Marques L, Alegria M, Becker AE, et al. Comparative prevalence, correlates of impairment, and service utilization for eating disorders across US ethnic groups: Implications for reducing ethnic disparities in health care access for eating disorders. Int J Eat Disord 2011;44(5):412–20.
58. Perez M, Ohrt TK, Hoek HW. Prevalence and treatment of eating disorders among Hispanics/Latino Americans in the United States. Curr Opin Psychiatry 2016;29(6):378–82.
59. Gorrell S, Murray SB. Eating disorders in males. Child Adolesc Psychiatr Clin N Am 2019;28(4):641–51.
60. Mahan LK, Raymond JL. Krause's food & the nutrition care process - E-Book (Krause's Food & Nutrition Therapy). 14th edition. Philadelphia, PA: Saunders; 2016. p. 930.
61. NIMH » Eating Disorders. Available at: https://www.nimh.nih.gov/health/topics/eating-disorders. Accessed March 8, 2022.
62. Eating Disorder Signs & Symptoms | Learn | NEDA. Available at: https://www.nationaleatingdisorders.org/warning-signs-and-symptoms. Accessed March 8, 2022.
63. Diabulimia | National Eating Disorders Association. Available at: https://www.nationaleatingdisorders.org/diabulimia-5. Accessed March 8, 2022.
64. Hill LS, Reid F, Morgan JF, et al. SCOFF, the development of an eating disorder screening questionnaire. Int J Eat Disord 2010;43(4):344–51.
65. Mond JM, Myers TC, Crosby RD, et al. Screening for eating disorders in primary care: EDE-Q versus SCOFF. Behav Res Ther 2008;46(5):612–22.
66. Penelo E, Villarroel AM, Portell M, et al. Eating Disorder Examination Questionnaire (EDE-Q). Eur J Psychol Assess 2012;28(1):76–83.
67. Gideon N, Hawkes N, Mond J, et al. Development and Psychometric Validation of the EDE-QS, a 12 Item Short Form of the Eating Disorder Examination Questionnaire (EDE-Q). PLoS One 2016;11(5):e0152744.
68. Puhl RM, Heuer CA. The stigma of obesity: a review and update. Obesity (Silver Spring) 2009;17(5):941–64.

69. Puhl R, Brownell KD. Bias, discrimination, and obesity. Obes Res 2001;9(12): 788–805.

70. Puhl RM, Phelan SM, Nadglowski J, et al. Overcoming weight bias in the management of patients with diabetes and obesity. Clin Diabetes 2016;34(1):44–50.

71. Alberga AS, Edache IY, Forhan M, et al. Weight bias and health care utilization: a scoping review. Prim Health Care Res Dev 2019;20:e116.

72. Healthcare Providers | UConn Rudd Center for Food Policy & Health. Available at: https://uconnruddcenter.org/research/weight-bias-stigma/healthcare-providers/. Accessed March 7, 2022.

73. Hager ER, Quigg AM, Black MM, et al. Development and validity of a 2-item screen to identify families at risk for food insecurity. Pediatrics 2010;126(1): e26–32.

74. Martin KS, Wu R, Wolff M, et al. A novel food pantry program: food security, self-sufficiency, and diet-quality outcomes. Am J Prev Med 2013;45(5):569–75.

75. Mishra S, Stierman B, Gahche JJ, et al. Dietary Supplement Use Among Adults: United States, 2017-2018. NCHS Data Brief 2021;(399):1–8.

76. Questions and Answers on Dietary Supplements | FDA. Available at: https://www.fda.gov/food/information-consumers-using-dietary-supplements/questions-and-answers-dietary-supplements. Accessed March 8, 2022.

77. Delichatsios HK, Hauser ME, Burgess JD, et al. Shared Medical Appointments: A Portal for Nutrition and Culinary Education in Primary Care-A Pilot Feasibility Project. Glob Adv Health Med 2015;4(6):22–6.

78. Sharma SV, McWhorter JW, Chow J, et al. Impact of a Virtual Culinary Medicine Curriculum on Biometric Outcomes, Dietary Habits, and Related Psychosocial Factors among Patients with Diabetes Participating in a Food Prescription Program. Nutrients 2021;13(12).

79. Little M, Rosa E, Heasley C, et al. Promoting healthy food access and nutrition in primary care: A systematic scoping review of food prescription programs. Am J Health Promot 2021. https://doi.org/10.1177/08901171211056584. 8901171211056584.

80. Rabaut LJ. Medically Tailored Meals as a Prescription for Treatment of Food-Insecure Type 2 Diabetics. J Patient Cent Res Rev 2019;6(2):179–83.

81. Downer S, Berkowitz SA, Harlan TS, et al. Food is medicine: actions to integrate food and nutrition into healthcare. BMJ 2020;369:m2482.

82. Berkowitz SA, Delahanty LM, Terranova J, et al. Medically Tailored Meal Delivery for Diabetes Patients with Food Insecurity: a Randomized Cross-over Trial. J Gen Intern Med 2019;34(3):396–404.

83. The Gaples Institute: A Fresh Approach to Nutrition and Lifestyle Education. Available at: https://www.gaplesinstitute.org/. Accessed April 8, 2022.

84. Healthy Kitchens, Healthy Lives. Available at: https://www.healthykitchens.org/. Accessed April 8, 2022.

85. Health meets Food: the Culinary Medicine Curriculum : CulinaryMedicine.org. Available at: https://culinarymedicine.org/. Accessed April 8, 2022.

86. National Board of Physician Nutrition Specialists. Available at: https://nbpns.org/. Accessed April 8, 2022.

87. La Puma J. What is culinary medicine and what does it do? Popul Health Manag 2016;19(1):1–3. https://doi.org/10.1089/pop.2015.0003.

Behavioral Approaches to Nutrition Counseling in the Primary Care Setting

Chinara Tate, PhD, RD

KEYWORDS

- Nutrition counseling • Nutrition care process • Motivational interviewing
- Cognitive behavioral therapy

KEY POINTS

- Evidence indicates that theory-based behavioral nutrition counseling strategies are effective in improving patient health outcomes.
- In the primary care setting, barriers to implementing behavioral nutrition counseling include lack of time, reimbursement, and perceived nutrition knowledge.
- Brief validated diet intake screeners and patient counseling applying core elements of theory-based strategies require little time, are low cost, and do not require in-depth nutrition knowledge.
- In practices where barriers are too great to implement any behavioral nutrition counseling strategies, singular recommendation to engage in normalized eating may have profound impact.

INTRODUCTION

Dietary factors have been identified as the single most significant risk factor for disability and premature death.[1] Minor dietary changes can result in marked improvement in patient health and quality of life. Despite the high prevalence of nutrition-related chronic conditions in the United States, only 12% of medical office visits include nutrition counseling.[2] In addition to increasing time constraints, many physicians report a lack of nutrition knowledge competence and low self-efficacy around dietary counseling.[3] In alignment with this finding, few medical schools offer students coursework dedicated to nutrition education and counseling with only 25% offering a nutrition-specific course. Far fewer schools achieve the 30 hours of nutrition education recommended by the National Academy of Sciences.[4]

Department of Psychiatry, Eating and Weight Disorders Program in Excellence, Icahn School of Medicine at Mount Sinai, One Gustave L. Levy Place, Box 1230, New York, NY 10029, USA
E-mail address: Chinara.Tate@mssm.edu

Med Clin N Am 106 (2022) 809–818
https://doi.org/10.1016/j.mcna.2022.06.002
medical.theclinics.com

Although time constraints are often cited as physicians' greatest barrier to providing nutrition counseling, it is evident that both nutrition education competency and cost are not far behind. Nutrition and behavioral counseling services are rarely reimbursed by insurance, although 15-minute intensive behavioral therapy obesity counseling is now offered to those with a Body Mass Index (BMI) $\geq$30 kg/m^2 as a Medicare obesity benefit by a licensed physician, only 1% of those eligible actually receive this service.[5] Although these challenges are significant, they are not entirely insurmountable. Here, we outline a number of low-burden steps clinicians can integrate into their workflow to include evidence-based approaches to behavioral nutrition counseling in patient care settings with limited resources and time.

DISCUSSION

In 2003, the American Dietetic Association adopted the nutrition care process (NCP) and model to standardize the structure and framework for providing individualized nutrition care across the dietetics profession.[6] Although some aspects of this process reach beyond the scope and resource limits of most primary care settings, the core principles and evidence-driven nutrition interventions derived from the NCP can be implemented with little cost, time, and resources.

The NCP is composed of four distinct steps: (1) nutrition assessment and reassessment, (2) nutrition diagnosis, (3) nutrition intervention, and (4) nutrition monitoring/evaluation.[7] Of these, nutrition assessment, intervention, and monitoring are the most appropriate, low-burden, and impactful ways physicians can improve patients dietary habits and related health outcomes. The sections below outline validated, evidence-supported ways primary care providers can incorporate meaningful nutrition care into daily practice.

Nutrition Care Process: Nutrition Assessment and Reassessment

In addition to routine biochemical data, anthropometric measurement, medical tests and procedures, the NCP-based nutrition assessment includes food or nutrition-related history.[7] Brief validated screeners such as the one below can be provided to patients in advance of their visit or while waiting to obtain an overview of each patient's dietary patterns and identify areas for further discussion around behavior change.

Starting the Conversation on Dietary Changes Screener

The 8-item validated "Starting the Conversation" food frequency screening tool can be used to quickly assess patients' daily eating habits and help the patient identify targets for change.[8] As discussed in detail below, nutrition interventions that are patient-driven and collaborative are more efficacious than unidirectional and confrontational recommendations. Further, placing the onus of reviewing and evaluating the screener on the patient reduces burden on the provider and narrows the focus of conversation to areas where the patient feels most confident and ready for change.

Although the screener is not diagnostic, it can be used to help inform and evaluate eating disorder risk and need for further assessment and referral. A diet low in fruits and vegetables and high in fast-food items, soda, desserts, and snack items may lead to discussion around amounts consumed, loss of control while eating, and possible need for BED evaluation. Conversely, a diet that is rich in fruits and vegetables but seems extremely restrictive in other areas may also warrant further discussion, evaluation, and possible referral to an eating disorders specialist.

(Scale developed by: the Center for Health Promotion and Disease Prevention, University of North Carolina at Chapel Hill, and North Carolina Prevention Partners)

Over the past few months:

		Less than 1 time	1–3 times	4 or more times
1.	How many times a week did you eat fast food meals or snacks?	☐ 0	☐ 1	☐ 2

		5 or more	3–4	2 or less
2.	How many servings of fruit did you eat each day?	☐ 0	☐ 1	☐ 2
3.	How many servings of vegetables did you eat each day?	☐ 0	☐ 1	☐ 2

		Less than 1	1–2	3 or more
4.	How many regular sodas or glasses of sweet tea did you drink each day?	☐ 0	☐ 1	☐ 2

		3 or more times	1–2 times	Less than 1 time
5.	How many times a week did you eat beans (like pinto or black beans), chicken, or fish?	☐ 0	☐ 1	☐ 2

		1 time or less	2–3 times	4 or more times
6.	How many times a week did you eat regular snack chips or crackers (not low-fat)?	☐ 0	☐ 1	☐ 2
7.	How many times a week did you eat desserts and other sweets (not the low-fat kind)?	☐ 0	☐ 1	☐ 2

		Very little	Some	A lot
8.	How much margarine, butter, or meat fat do you use to season vegetables or put on potatoes, bread, or corn?	☐ 0	☐ 1	☐ 2

SUMMARY SCORE (sum of all items): _____

NCP: Nutrition Intervention

Nutrition Care Process: Nutrition Intervention

Evidence suggests that theory-informed nutrition interventions are more effective in promoting behavior change than those that are not informed by theory.[9] More specifically, nutrition interventions based on behavioral theory, cognitive behavioral theory, and social cognitive theory have demonstrated consistent and significant effectiveness in dietary behavior modification and health outcomes.[10] When feasible, theory-based nutrition counseling techniques can more effectively help assess each patient's current motivation for dietary change and beliefs around implementing those changes and identify additional supports to help patients begin to make and sustain those changes long term. Two well established and effective evidence-based nutrition counseling strategies include motivational interviewing (MI) and cognitive behavioral therapy (CBT). Importantly, both of these counseling approaches place patients at the center of behavior change planning and problem-solving, making the providers' nutrition knowledge less essential to intervention delivery and effective counseling.

Motivational Interviewing

MI is a patient-centered and provider-guided approach aimed at helping patients increase their commitment to, motivation for, and confidence around behavior change based on their personal values and goals. Several studies indicate that MI significantly improves cardiovascular health, glycemic control, percentage of energy intake from fat, fruit and vegetable intake, and weight loss.[11–18]

The primary role of the provider in MI is to present questions that help the patient identify their motives for change, current barriers, and uncover potential ways to address those barriers based on lived experience and perceived resources. Central to MI is a communication style that uses a mix of open-ended questions, affirmations, reflections, and summaries to express non-judgment, collaboration, respect, acceptance, and compassion.[19] Some examples of these are included as follows:

Open-Ended Questions
- What are your primary health concerns?
- How is your health currently affecting you?
- How would making this change make your life better?

Affirmations
- It is clear you are committed to leading a healthier lifestyle.
- You have done an excellent job of identifying your primary motivations for change.

Reflections
- I am hearing that you notice you are less likely to eat past fullness when you do not go into a meal extremely hungry—is that accurate?

Summaries
- From our conversation today you sound very committed to improving your health. Now that you have outlined some of the ways your life and health might improve by consuming more fruits and vegetables, it sounds as if you are interested in exploring how you can incorporate more of these in your diet. Earlier you mentioned that because you're working long hours at your desk, you can only make a change that is quick and easy.

In terms of structure and sequence, MI can be broadly divided into four core processes:

1. Engage
   - After providing a warm and friendly greeting, ask open-ended questions to build rapport and assess what the patient's primary health concerns are.
2. Focus
   - After establishing rapport, invite the patient to focus on a specific topic and lead with an open-ended question such as "Given you have expressed increased difficulty going up the stairs at home, is there a specific change you have thought about making?" This narrows the focus of the conversation to the patients' primary concern while also placing them at the lead in problem-solving.
3. Evoke
   - If a patient expresses hesitancy around making change, ask open-ended questions aimed at evoking and supporting change talk such as "What might be some benefits of making this change?" and "How might these changes improve your daily life?"
4. Plan

- Empower and guide patients toward developing their own plan and strategies for implementing change by asking questions such as "How might you go about making that change?"

Cognitive Behavioral Therapy

CBT is based on two well established and tested behavior change theories—behavioral theory and cognitive behavioral theory.[20] Evidence suggests that CBT is a highly effective behavioral nutrition counseling strategy, particularly when used in conjunction with MI. To date, there are more than 20 RCT studies providing evidence for CBTs effectiveness in modifying specific dietary behaviors (eg, increased fruit and vegetable intake) toward weight management, reduced diabetes, and cardiovascular risk.[20] The National Heart, Lung, and Blood Institute and the American Diabetes Association both recommend behavioral therapy for weight management.[21,22] CBT examines both external and internal factors to help patients explore, identify, and analyze how their patterns of thinking, feeling, and acting interact and may be at odds with their expressed goals. The key strategies for CBT-based nutrition counseling include:

- Self-monitoring: This patient-directed process involves recording thoughts, emotions, dietary behaviors, physical activities, and health measurements (eg, blood sugar, blood pressure). The patient's self-monitoring record is then reviewed with a provider to identify triggers and patterns to assist in problem-solving and goal-setting.
- Problem-solving: Like MI, CBT also encourages a collaborative approach in problem-solving that involves identifying barriers, brainstorming potential solutions, and examining the pros and cons of potential solutions before implementation.
- Goal-setting: This central component of CBT involves helping patients set goals that are specific, measurable, achievable/realistic, time-bound (SMART goals). Monitoring and documenting patient progress toward long- and short-term goals is essential to effectiveness.
- Rewards: A systematic plan for receipt of patient-identified rewards may be used to incentivize specific dietary behavior changes.
- Social support: A patient's network of family, friends, colleagues, and health professionals are all key components of social support requisite for encouragement, emotional support, and information to support behavior change.

Cognitive Behavioral Therapy and Normalized Eating

In addition to diet-related chronic disease outcomes, evidence supports the use of CBT in eating disorder treatment of those with anorexia (AN), bulimia (BN), binge eating disorder (BED), and eating disorder not otherwise specified (NOS).[23] Before engaging in any other dietary changes, patients presenting with eating disorders are advised to establish a pattern of regular eating including three meals and two to three planned snacks with no more than a 4-hour interval between.[23–26] In patients who are subthreshold for eating disorder diagnosis or engage in disturbed eating behaviors (restrictive eating, cyclical dieting, and bingeing), normalized eating may also be beneficial in improving health outcomes.

A Brief Approach to Behavioral Nutrition Counseling in Primary Care Settings:

1. Engage: Build rapport with warm empathy and active listening

2. Focus: Have the patient review their "Start the conversation" screener and identify one dietary change the feel motivated to make.

3. Evoke: Ask the patient to identify one to two benefits associated with this change.

4. Plan: Ask the patient to set a specific measurable goal around this change and write it down.

5. Recommend Normalized Eating: If there is an evidence of disturbed eating patterns (dietary restraint, restriction, cyclical dieting, and bingeing) propose that before implementing any other dietary changes they try to eat at regular intervals including three meals and two to three snacks as a first step.

6. Enlist Support: Assess a patient's social support structure. Refer to a specialist as needed for additional support.

Additional Behavior Change Theory Models and Approaches

Although rigorous study and evidence for the effectiveness of other behavior change theories in nutrition-related health outcomes is lacking, these may serve as meaningful approaches to address gaps in MI and CBT, conceptualize patient's readiness for change, and provide patients with additional support.

Transtheoretical (Stages of Change) Model

In addition to assessing dietary intake, it is important to assess a patient's readiness for change. The transtheoretical model, also known as the stages of change model, posits that patients cycle through five distinct stages of readiness for change that include:

1. Precontemplation
2. Contemplation
3. Preparation
4. Action
5. Maintenance

In nutrition counseling, the provider is tasked with both assessing which stage the patient is presently at and using four key strategies to help the patient move to the next stage.[27] These strategies include (1) consciousness raising, (2) environmental reevaluation, (3) helping relationships, and (4) self-evaluation. The role of the provider in this model is to help the patient move from one stage to the next toward taking and sustaining action by providing education and/or educational resources (consciousness raising); discussing the role of the patient's physical and social environment on their diet, physical activity, and coping strategies (environmental reevaluation); identifying social support structures to seek and accept support (helping relationships); appraising alignment between patient values and behavior change goals (self-reevaluation); and evaluating pros, cons, and perceived barriers behavior change.[28]

Self-Determination Theory

Despite efforts to outline the benefits of behavior change, address perceived barriers, and enlist support, low motivation to change is frequently cited as a major obstacle in behavioral nutrition counseling. Self-determination theory (SDT) places motivation in the framework of internal and external motivators. Internal motivators are based on personal values and interest, eliciting intrinsic feelings of reward (eg, enjoyment). External motivators include outside factors that motivate the patient to engage in behavior change such as desire to avoid conflict with a family member, a contingency for not complying, and tangible rewards for engaging in the behavior. The role of the provider using SDT is to help identify whether the patient is more internally or externally motivated, draw on effective motivators to elicit behavior change and ultimately help the more externally motivated patient internalize changes toward internal motivation and greater autonomy (self-determination).[29]

Social Cognitive Theory/Ecological Models

Social cognitive theory underscores the importance and interaction between the patient and their environment.[30,31] In the context of nutrition counseling, this model takes into account the impact environmental factors such as food availability, affordability, and accessibility may have on a patient's choices and behaviors. These environmental resources and barriers are observed at multiple levels and include the patient's interpersonal relationships, family, community, and city. In the context of often environmental factors that are not immediately mutable (eg, community and city levels), Social cognitive theory highlights two major factors as central promoting behavior change: (1) self-efficacy and (2) outcome expectations. Self-efficacy is defined as the degree to which the patient believes that they can change or maintain a specific behavior regardless of external circumstances.[32] Evidence suggests that high self-efficacy is associated with better treatment outcomes.[33] A patient's self-efficacy may be aligned with their perceived or actual personal knowledge, skills, resources, or environmental supports.[34] Providers may help patients increase self-efficacy by directing them to resources to heighten their knowledge and skills. Outcome expectations are defined as the anticipated positive or negative consequences the patient believes they will experience as a result of engaging in a behavior. By reviewing outcome expectations with the patient the provider may help them evaluate whether these expectations are accurate or warrant modification.

SUMMARY

In primary health care settings, time and resources are seldom adequate to deliver comprehensive behavioral nutrition counseling to patients at high risk for diet-related chronic conditions such as diabetes, cardiovascular disease, and some cancers. Although MI and CBT offer a theory-based framework and strategy for using evidence-based nutrition guidance, primary care providers often lack training and bandwidth to deliver such services consistently, if at all.

A more plausible middle path may be to apply core MI and CBT principles with one singular recommendation toward normalized eating. This patient-centered collaborative approach may not only reduce resistance to change but enable patients to begin with one important evidence-based step that is recommended to improve eating habits before any changes are made to dietary content—eating on a regular schedule. On screening and evaluation, referral and follow-up with a registered dietician and/or eating disorders specialist may be indicated to support or augment the primary care practitioners' efforts. Normalized eating is often the first recommendation made for patients with BED, AN, and BN. Although many patients may not meet formal The Diagnostic and Statistical Manual of Mental Disorders, Fifth Edition (DSM-V) criteria for these conditions, they may not be able to make the dietary change they have identified if they do not build a habit of eating on a regular consistent basis.

By engaging patients in brief but meaningful components of theory-based behavioral nutrition counseling in a manner that is nonjudgmental, empathetic and collaborative primary care practitioners may not only help patients initiate change they may provide them with the tools and foundational trust needed to enlist additional resources toward long-lasting change in their dietary habits and health outcomes.

Technological advances in mobile apps may also support primary care providers' efforts toward patients' behavioral nutrition modification.[35–38] Efforts to refine a precision medicine approach using machine learning and psychosocial-behavioral phenotyping offer great promise for highly tailored yet more broadly accessible behavioral nutrition recommendations, resources, and support.[39]

CLINICS CARE POINTS

- Patient nutrition intake can be assessed rapidly with a brief validated screener in office or electronically before arrival.
- In depth nutrition knowledge is not required to deliver effective strategies for behavioral nutrition counseling.
- MI and CBT are patient-centered processes that ask them to identify dietary habits they want to change, barriers they may encounter, and possible solutions to meet their goals.
- Avoid a confrontational approach to nutrition counseling as this can shut patients down and is unlikely to be effective.
- Evidence supports a nonjudgmental, collaborative approach to behavioral nutritional counseling.
- Normalized eating is recommended for all patients seeking to make dietary changes and can serve as a pivotal step in attaining their nutrition-related goals.

ACKNOWLEDGMENTS

This article is presented with dedication to and in memory of the author's late father, Gregory Stephen Tate, and late beloved and dear friend, Jason O. Forde.

DISCLOSURE

There are no commercial or financial conflicts of interest to disclose.

REFERENCES

1. Mokdad AH, Ballestros K, Echko M, et al. The state of US health, 1990-2016: Burden of Diseases, Injuries, and Risk Factors Among US States. JAMA 2018; 319:1444–72.
2. Healthy people 2020. PsycEXTRA Dataset; 2010. https://doi.org/10.1037/e589962012-001.
3. Hutchinson E, Catlin M, Andrilla CHA, et al. Barriers to primary care physicians prescribing buprenorphine. Ann Fam Med 2014;12:128–33.
4. Adams KM, Kohlmeier M, Zeisel SH. Nutrition education in U.S. medical schools: latest update of a national survey. Acad Med 2010;85:1537–42.
5. Batsis JA, Bynum JPW. Uptake of the centers for medicare and medicaid obesity benefit: 2012-2013. Obesity 2016;24:1983–8.
6. Lacey K, Pritchett E. Nutrition care process and model: ADA adopts road map to quality care and outcomes management. J Am Diet Assoc 2003;103:1061–72.
7. Nutrition care process. Available at: https://www.eatrightpro.org/practice/quality-management/nutrition-care-process. Assessed May 14, 2022.

8. Paxton AE, Strycker LA, Toobert DJ, et al. Starting the conversation performance of a brief dietary assessment and intervention tool for health professionals. Am J Prev Med 2011;40:67–71.

9. Michie S, Abraham C, Whittington C, et al. Effective techniques in healthy eating and physical activity interventions: a meta-regression. Health Psychol 2009;28: 690–701.

10. Rigby RR, Mitchell LJ, Hamilton K, et al. The use of behavior change theories in dietetics practice in primary health care: a systematic review of randomized controlled trials. J Acad Nutr Diet 2020;120:1172–97.

11. VanWormer JJ, Boucher JL. Motivational interviewing and diet modification: a review of the evidence. Diabetes Educ 2004;30(404–6):408–10, 414–6 passim.

12. Brug J, Spikmans F, Aartsen C, et al. Training dietitians in basic motivational interviewing skills results in changes in their counseling style and in lower saturated fat intakes in their patients. J Nutr Educ Behav 2007;39:8–12.

13. Macdonell K, Brogan K, Naar-King S, et al. A pilot study of motivational interviewing targeting weight-related behaviors in overweight or obese African American adolescents. J Adolesc Health 2012;50:201–3.

14. Bean MK, Powell P, Quinoy A, et al. Motivational interviewing targeting diet and physical activity improves adherence to paediatric obesity treatment: results from the MI Values randomized controlled trial. Pediatr Obes 2015;10:118–25.

15. Miller ST, Oates VJ, Brooks MA, et al. Preliminary efficacy of group medical nutrition therapy and motivational interviewing among obese African American women with type 2 diabetes: a pilot study. J Obes 2014;2014:345941.

16. Armstrong MJ, Mottershead TA, Ronksley PE, et al. Motivational interviewing to improve weight loss in overweight and/or obese patients: a systematic review and meta-analysis of randomized controlled trials. Obes Rev 2011;12:709–23.

17. Thompson DR. Motivational interviewing: a useful approach to improving cardiovascular health? J Clin Nurs 2011;20:1236–44.

18. Channon SJ, Huws-Thomas MV, Rollnick S, et al. A multicenter randomized controlled trial of motivational interviewing in teenagers with diabetes. Diabetes Care 2007;30:1390–5.

19. Miller WR, Rollnick S. Motivational interviewing: helping people change. Guilford Press; 2012.

20. Spahn JM, Reeves RS, Keim KS, et al. State of the evidence regarding behavior change theories and strategies in nutrition counseling to facilitate health and food behavior change. J Am Diet Assoc 2010;110:879–91.

21. Managing overweight and obesity in adults: systematic evidence review from the obesity expert panel. Available at: https://www-nhlbi-nih-gov.eresources.mssm.edu/health-topics/managing-overweight-obesity-in-adults. Assessed May 28, 2022.

22. Bantle JP, Wylie-Rosett J, Albright AL, et al. Nutrition recommendations and interventions for diabetes: a position statement of the American Diabetes Association. Diabetes Care 2008;31(Suppl 1):S61–78.

23. Murphy R, Straebler S, Cooper Z, et al. Cognitive behavioral therapy for eating disorders. Psychiatr Clin North Am 2010;33:611–27.

24. Shah N, Passi V, Bryson S, et al. Patterns of eating and abstinence in women treated for bulimia nervosa. Int J Eat Disord 2005;38:330–4.

25. Ellison JM, Simonich HK, Wonderlich SA, et al. Meal patterning in the treatment of bulimia nervosa. Eat Behav 2016;20:39–42.

26. Sivyer K, Allen E, Cooper Z, et al. Mediators of change in cognitive behavior therapy and interpersonal psychotherapy for eating disorders: A secondary analysis

of a transdiagnostic randomized controlled trial. Int J Eat Disord 2020;53: 1928–40.

27. Prochaska JO, Diclemente CC. Toward a comprehensive model of change. Treating addictive behaviors, 3–27. US: Springer; 1986.

28. Prochaska JO, Velicer WF. The transtheoretical model of health behavior change. Am J Health Promot 1997;12:38–48.

29. Deci EL, Ryan RM. Self-determination theory. In: Higgins E, editor. Handbook of theories of social psychology. Thousand Oaks, CA: Sage Publications Ltd; vol. 1. 2012. p. 416–36.

30. Baranowski T, Cullen KW, Nicklas T, et al. Are current health behavioral change models helpful in guiding prevention of weight gain efforts? Obes Res 2003; 11(Suppl):23S–43S.

31. Anderson ES, Winett RA, Wojcik JR. Self-regulation, self-efficacy, outcome expectations, and social support: social cognitive theory and nutrition behavior. Ann Behav Med 2007;34:304–12.

32. Conner M, Norman P. *EBOOK*: Predicting and changing health behaviour: research and practice with social cognition models. UK): McGraw-Hill Education; 2015.

33. King DK, Glasgow RE, Toobert DJ, et al. Self-efficacy, problem solving, and social-environmental support are associated with diabetes self-management behaviors. Diabetes Care 2010;33:751–3.

34. Bandura, A. Self-efficacy: The exercise of control. 604, (1997).

35. Rohde A, Duensing A, Dawczynski C, et al. An App to Improve Eating Habits of Adolescents and Young Adults (Challenge to Go): Systematic Development of a Theory-Based and Target Group-Adapted Mobile App Intervention. JMIR Mhealth Uhealth 2019;7:e11575.

36. Villinger K, Wahl DR, Boeing H, et al. The effectiveness of app-based mobile interventions on nutrition behaviours and nutrition-related health outcomes: A systematic review and meta-analysis. Obes Rev 2019;20:1465–84.

37. Kankanhalli A, Shin J, Oh H. Mobile-based interventions for dietary behavior change and health outcomes: scoping review. JMIR Mhealth Uhealth 2019;7: e11312.

38. Coughlin SS, Whitehead M, Sheats JQ, et al. Smartphone applications for promoting healthy diet and nutrition: a literature review. Jacobs J Food Nutr 2015; 2:021.

39. Burgermaster M, Rodriguez VA. Psychosocial-behavioral phenotyping: a novel precision health approach to modeling behavioral, psychological, and social determinants of health using machine learning. Ann Behav Med 2022. https://doi. org/10.1093/abm/kaac012.

Nutrition Guidelines for Improved Clinical Care

Ted Wilson, PhD[a],*, Adrianne Bendich, PhD, FASN[b]

KEYWORDS

- Diet • Nutrition • Essential nutrients • Hydration • Alcohol
- Recommended dietary COVID-19

KEY POINTS

- Nutrition receives little attention in health-care training but nutrition understanding is essential.
- Specific vitamins, minerals, and certain other nutrients are essential for health.
- The liquids that are central to our essential hydration can also influence dietary health.
- Understanding how to use the dietary guidelines and nutrition facts labeling can improve nutritional status and the consumption of a healthy diet.
- COVID-19 has altered access to nutritious foods for millions and increased awareness of the importance of diet and immune function.

INTRODUCTION

Suboptimal nutrition is the central pillar supporting most clinically relevant diseases; in this regard, observational data suggest that diet may be a factor in 45% of all deaths due to heart disease, stroke, and type 2 diabetes.[1] Indeed preventive nutrition is central to US programs for economically disadvantaged populations such as the women, infants, and children (WIC) and other prenatal programs that help to reduce the risk of preterm birth, infant diseases, and birth defects.[2,3] Paradoxically, in a 2008 to 2009 survey, only 26% of US Medical Schools required even a single course in nutrition and on average only 19.6 hours of instruction in nutrition were completed during the 4 years of training.[4] A more recent review confirms that the number of hours spent in medical school devoted to nutrition is about 19.[5] Moreover, as of this writing, the Accreditation Council for Graduate Medical Education has no requirement for nutrition education during residency or fellowship training and/or advanced specialty training including gastroenterology and cardiology.[5]

[a] Department of Biology, Winona State University, Rm 232, Pasteur Hall, Winona, MN 55987, USA; [b] Springer/Nature Nutrition and Health Book Series Editor, retired, 8765 Via Brilliante Wellington, FL 33411, USA
* Corresponding author. Department of Biology, Winona State University, Winona, MN 55987.
E-mail address: twilson@winona.edu

Med Clin N Am 106 (2022) 819–836
https://doi.org/10.1016/j.mcna.2022.04.007
0025-7125/22/© 2022 Elsevier Inc. All rights reserved.

One objective of this article is to provide physicians with the basics of dietary requirements including a clear description of the essential nutrients that all humans require to live regardless of the growing cultural dietary melting pot that the clinician encounters and attempts to interpret. The article includes novel topics of patient interest, including the critical importance of hydration and the many types of liquids available today. Educating patients in a convincing manner to encourage them to choose the best evidence-based path to good nutrition has always been troublesome for both the patient and the physician. The reality is that in a relatively heterogeneous world of many different culturally based food choices and eating plans, there are many preconceptions about what constitutes a "healthy balanced diet and/or healthy food." Moreover, the data-based field of nutritional genetics ensures that there cannot be any one single best path for every single patient.

Clinicians are often left to make nutrition recommendations based on those from many different "professional" organizations, whose recommendations are not always in agreement; the influence of nonprofessional opinions expressed in blogs, websites, and Television (TV) further clouds the clarity of clinical suggestions. This article provides the clinician with important data-based key information (morsels) to better understand the twenty-first century nutrition guidelines and to advise patients with tools to implement dietary change based on facts and data. Thus, the article contains a historic review of the development of National guidelines and recommendations from the US National Academy of Sciences (NAS), the United States Department of Agriculture (USDA), Centers for Disease Control (CDC) and Food and Drug Administration (FDA) to better help explain the current status of nutrition and dietary guidelines and food product labeling.

Finally, Coronavirus disease 2019 (COVID-19) has altered the public's perception of the importance of nutrition for a healthy immune system. The article concludes with an up-to-date look at the interface between obesity, diabetes, and other examples of malnutrition and a description of how nutritional status is a major factor associated with in increased risk of severe COVID-19-related medical complications.

Links Between Diet and Disease: Essential Nutrients

Vitamins and minerals

Links between diet and disease have been recorded as early as 1500 BC when ancient Egyptians ate liver (rich in vitamin A) as a cure for night blindness.[6] The term, "scurvy," meaning swollen mouth, was documented in the Middle Ages. Certainly, the importance of isolating citrus fruits to prevent scurvy was a major breakthrough in the eighteenth century.[7] However, it was not until the early years of the twentieth century that the 11 individual vitamins were isolated and their chemical formulas were determined. By 1948, all of the vitamins were discovered and chemically identified and are summarized in **Table 1**.[8] Thus, we remain in the discovery period for how these essential nutrients (defined as molecules that cannot be synthesized by our own bodies and are essential for life) affect our health as well as our responses to deficiencies, diseases, and injury.

Vitamins are not the only essential nutrients for humans. By definition, all mineral elements that are found in the human body are essential as no one has yet synthesized an element. There are 2 classifications of essential mineral elements, major and trace. The major mineral elements include calcium, phosphorus, potassium, sodium, and magnesium. The trace elements include sulfur, iron, chlorine, cobalt, copper, zinc, manganese, molybdenum, iodine, and selenium. Each of the 15 minerals has their own constellation of deficiency symptoms such as iron deficiency anemia and osteoporosis due to calcium deficiency (**Table 2**).[9] We are still learning about the essentiality

Table 1
Vitamins and their key deficiency disease symptoms. Fat soluble vitamins are colored red; B vitamins are colored blue

Vitamin	Deficiency Symptom(s)
A (retinol)	Night blindness, xerophthalmia
Thiamin (B1)	Beriberi, polyneuropathy, Wernicke's encephalopathy
Riboflavin (B2)	Glossitis, dermatitis
Niacin	Pellagra, diarrhea, mental disturbance
B6 (pyridoxine)	Macrocytic anemia, depression convulsions
B12 (cobalamin)	Macrocytic anemia, peripheral neuritis, spinal cord degeneration
Biotin	Dermatitis, axorexia, muscular pain
Pantothenic acid	Nervous and intestinal disorders
Folic acid	Anemia, macrocytic anemia
C (ascorbic acid)	Scurvy, sore gums, capillary bleeding
D (cholecalciferol)	Rickets, bone deformity, tetany
E (tocopherol)	Hemolytic anemia, neuromuscular dysfunction
K (phylloquinone)	Decreased blood clotting, bleeding

Modified From: Vitamin Intake and Health, edited by S.K. Gaby, A. Bendich, V. N. Singh, L. J. Machlin, 1991, pp 1-16.[8]

of trace minerals as can be seen by the inclusion of chromium for the first time as essential nutrient in the 2001 edition of the US Dietary Reference Intakes (DRIs).[10]

Essential fats

With the clear findings that dietary deficiencies of vitamins were causing serious health issues including death, there was a strong impetus to determine if there were other essential nutrients required in the human diet. Clinical nutrition researchers in the 1930s were looking for the link between signs of deficiencies associated with the development of scaly skin, reproductive failure, growth failure, and kidney degeneration in animal models. They identified 2 more essential nutrients: the fatty acids, linoleic acid, an omega-6 fatty acid and linolenic acid, an omega-3 fatty acid. Both are the building blocks of all other fatty acids that can be synthesized in the body to varying degrees. The fatty acids are required for formation of the lipid bilayer around every cell, the synthesis of hormones, growth factors, prostaglandins and other immune factors,

Table 2
Common minerals and their associated deficiency symptoms

Mineral	Deficiency Symptom(s)
Iron	Iron deficiency anemia
Iodine	Infancy—congenital hypothyroidism with potential cognitive loses Adults—thyroid goiter
Zinc	Acrodermatitis enteropathica, growth retardation, hypogeusia
Magnesium	Tremor, muscle spasm, nystagmus, seizures
Selenium	Keshan disease—cardiomyopathy
Calcium	Osteoporosis

Modified From: Stephenson, T., Sanctuary, M. R. Passerrello, C.W. Human Nutrition: Science for Healthy Living. McGraw-Hill, 2022.[9]

and many more molecules necessary for cell-to-cell communication.[11] Moreover, the fat-soluble vitamins (A, E, D, and K) as well as vitamin precursors, such as fat-soluble beta-carotene (the major source of vitamin A) are best absorbed when there is fat in the diet. Even though it was well accepted that humans require consumption of these 2 essential fatty acids, even in the 1989 recommended dietary allowance (RDA) report for many reasons the subcommittee had not established an RDA for n-3 or n-6 poly-unsaturated fatty acids.[12] This was because essential fatty acid deficiency had been observed exclusively in patients with medical problems affecting fat intake or absorption.

Essential amino acids

In addition to the 11 vitamins, 15 minerals and 2 fatty acids, there are 9 more essen-tial nutrients for humans and these are 9 amino acids: phenylalanine, valine, threo-nine, tryptophan, methionine, leucine, isoleucine, lysine, and histidine. Amino acids are the key components of all proteins.[13] Certain amino acids, including some of the essential ones, have unique functions independent of protein synthesis. In total, there are 21 amino acids, 12 of which can be synthesized by humans and 9 that must be consumed. The major natural source of essential amino acids is protein, mainly animal protein for balanced amnio acid delivery. There are protein sources that do not contain all of the essential amino acids and if humans, especially infants and growing children consume protein sources that do not contain all of the essential amino acids, they will not thrive. As a result they will lose weight, develop edema, be lethargic and can lose cognitive abilities, even if there is only one of the 9 amino acids absent in the diet of a young child or an adult. Deficiency symptoms manifest them-selves even when the subjects are unaware, and during a pronounced negative ni-trogen balance, problems with appetite, extreme fatigue, and nervous irritability can develop.[13] The essential amino acids are discussed in the text of the 1989 RDA; however, recommendations are made for total protein intake not individual essential amino acids.[12]

Carbohydrates

Carbohydrates represent a clinical paradox with respect to their being essential in the healthy human diet, but not an essential "nutrient" based on the classic definition. Car-bohydrates consist of monosaccharides (ie, glucose), disaccharides (ie, lactose) and polysaccharides (ie, starch, glycogen and plant-fiber). Polysaccharides such as starch in a cracker are readily metabolized, whereas fiber is a carbohydrate and is not metab-olized by the digestive enzymes available in the human gut.

Although adult humans have a carbohydrate RDA of 130 g/d, there are examples of populations existing on a virtually carbohydrate-free diet. The historic Inuit Eski-mos of Greenland almost never developed Cardiovascular disease (CVD) or dia-betes, and relied almost completely on a meat-based diet with little or no carbohydrate intake before the introduction of Western diets and diseases.[14] They lived a very physically active lifestyle and survived (thrived) on the fat and protein in meat and used gluconeogenic amino acids from that meat to create the glucose required for neural function. However, between 1951 and 1961, the Inuit of Canada had a life expectancy at birth of 37 years, which was 33 years lower than the Cana-dian average,[15] and it is possibly not surprising the possible cardiovascular disease benefits of their low-carbohydrate diet may reflect that these persons simply did not live long enough to develop cardiovascular disease. Recently, there has been increased interest in carbohydrate-free diets. However, long-term human random-ized control trials that examine the safety of a carbohydrate-free diet do not exist, and most studies of low-carbohydrate diets (aka Atkins. Ketogenic, Low Carb Paleo, and so forth) are neither double blind nor last longer than a year.

Undeniably, consumption of large amounts of refined dietary carbohydrates for long periods have been consistently associated with a variety of diseases including obesity, diabetes, cancer, and cardiovascular disease. Paradoxically, persons living in the absence of dietary fiber and whole grains are also more likely to develop diseases such as colon cancer and cardiovascular disease. However, because production of a pound of meat requires at least 10 lbs of grain, it has been proposed that the dietary carbohydrates will need to become an ever more essential part of the human diet if we hope to feed our planet in an environmentally sustainable fashion.[16]

Increased intakes of carbohydrates have been linked with increased risk of obesity and an upper safe limit has not been uniformly agreed on. Increased obesity and fatness are well-known risk factors for cardiovascular disease and early death. Body mass index (BMI) is often used to assess fatness or whether a patient is effectively making dietary changes to facilitate improvements in adiposity. BMI is defined as the body mass (weight) divided by the square of the body height or weight in pounds divided by height in inches squared times 703. BMI categorizes adults as underweight (less than 18.5 kg/m^2), normal weight (18.5–24.9), overweight (25–29.9), and obese (30 or more). The CDC growth charts predict BMI/age for children ages 2 to 20 years that help track growth and changing nutrient intake from birth to adulthood (http://www.cdc.gov/growthcharts).[17] Although BMI assessment is simple and easy to perform, it may only be predictive of obesity as little as 50% of the time.[18] Although BMI is predictive of overall mortality, it is not perfect, and personal fitness level (eg, Vo$_2$ max) is more reliable for predicting health and overall mortality, as well as more expensive.[19] Changes in nutrition and exercise fitness are not always reflective of changes in BMI. There is often a clinical misunderstanding when determining if a patient is successfully changing their diet across a treatment regimen. Other articles in this series provide greater details regarding the utility of BMI for the assessment of nutrition behavioral change.

Water and other liquid sources of hydration

Water intake is necessary for human survival. Everyday physiologic functions, such as perspiration, urination, and healthy bowel movements, diminish the body's water content, and therefore, water intake must be sufficient daily to account for these losses. For adults who are not exercising, the daily adequate intake level for women is 2.7 L (91 ounces 11.3 cups) and 3.7 L (125 ounces or 15.6 cups) from all food and beverage sources.[20] Water needs can also be estimated to be 35 to 45 mL/kg/d, and during exercise, needs increase by about 1 mL water for each calorie of oxidized energy used during exercise.[21] Care must be taken when estimating human water requirements because of the tremendous variations in human body weight, levels of activity, and basic health (water loss due to sweating or diarrhea), and the water content of the food consumed.

Although water is the most common substance on Earth, access to drinkable, clean water remains a major concern in many regions of the world and even in the United States with respect to the problem in Flint Michigan's struggle with tap-water lead contamination.[22] Generally, tap water is safe in the United States and the best source of water, readily available, and the most cost-effective; for this reason, clinicians should promote it in the clinical setting.

Green tea consumption has been linked to reducing the risk of cancer[23] and cardiovascular disease.[24] A recent green tea meta-analysis by Wang and colleagues suggests that the protective relationship is strongest for green tea and slightly protective for black tea.[25] Green tea consumption was found to be particularly protective against all cause mortality for those who had a prior stroke or myocardial infarct.[26]

Coffee consumption is considered safe and may provide several health benefits. Coffee intake may even be protective against the development of hypertension in comparison to noncoffee drinkers.[27] Cardiovascular disease risk is lowest for those consuming 3 to 5 cups of caffeinated coffee per day, with consumption of more than 6 cups/d remaining relatively neutral for CVD risk.[28] Moderate coffee consumption is inversely significantly associated with CVD risk, with the lowest CVD risk at 3 to 5 cups/d, and heavy coffee consumption was not associated with elevated CVD risk. In addition, recent evidence suggests that coffee consumption may be beneficial for preventing type 2 diabetes,[29] a condition commonly associated with cardiovascular disease. Caffeinated coffee is also associated with improved cognitive function in persons aged older than 60 years, although the effect was not strong for consumers of decaffeinated coffee.[30] Most epidemiologic studies show the absence of any appreciable association between coffee intake and most common neoplasms; indeed, an inverse relationship between coffee consumption and colorectal cancer risk may exist.[31]

Dairy milk has long been recognized as a way to improve calcium intake and bone health, especially when it is fortified with vitamin D. The high-calcium content in milk and its lipid content, which improves absorption of lipid-soluble vitamins, make it ideal as a medium for vitamin D fortification. Milk is also an excellent source of potassium, magnesium, and protein. The Dietary Approaches to Stop Hypertension (DASH) study suggested that low-fat dairy consumption may reduce blood pressure.[32] Milk does not seem to affect overall mortality and may reduce the risk of cardiovascular disease, an effect that is probably stronger for low-fat milk.[33]

Nondairy milk is often preferred by patients who choose to not consume dairy milk products for a variety of reasons that include lactose intolerance, dietary preferences (vegetarian), taste, environmental sustainability, or health concerns that may or may not be supported by clinical evidence. Plant-based milks derived from almond, palm, oats, rice, and other plants have been widely accepted among consumers, with soy-milk remaining the most popular. Plant-based milks were estimated to represent upward of 13% of the total US milk market in 2020.[34] Although the nutritional content of dairy (cow) milk products is relatively consistent, nutritional contents of plant-based milks are more variable making any one clinical recommendation for all plant-based milk more difficult; the differing degree of nutritional supplementation further complicates the use of any single recommendation,[35] especially for children.[36]

Fruit juices are a popular way to increase fruit consumption because of their widespread accessibility, ease of storage, modest cost, and for hedonistic reasons (taste). The USDA recommendations at MyPlate suggest using 100% fruit juice as equivalent to a fruit serving for the purpose of the plate.[37] The energy content of apple juice and orange juice (110 kcal/240 mL serving) is about 6% higher than that of cola drinks. The energy content of white grape juice is even higher, around 150 kcal/240 mL. Overconsumption of fruit or vegetable juices can lead to excess carbohydrate intake and weight gain, so caution should always be given in the clinical setting.

Sugar sweetened beverages (SSBs) intake assessed by the The National Health and Nutrition Examination Survey (NHANES) 2005 to 2006 data set for adolescents aged 13 to 19 years averaged 242 kcal/d of soft and fruit drinks that represented about 17% of daily caloric intake.[38] Adult and adolescent obesities are increasing in the United States but the exact reason for this is probably multifactorial, although Sugar sweetened beverages (SSB) consumption is probably one contributing factor. In adults, consumption of SSB is positively and tightly correlated with weight gain and

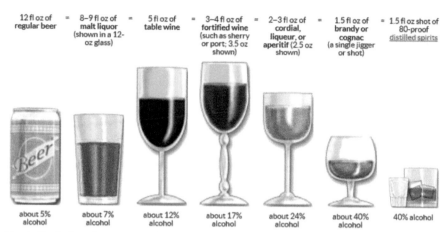

| 12 fl oz of regular beer | = | 8–9 fl oz of malt liquor (shown in a 12-oz glass) | = | 5 fl oz of table wine | = | 3–4 fl oz of fortified wine (such as sherry or port; 3.5 oz shown) | = | 2–3 fl oz of cordial, liqueur, or aperitif (2.5 oz shown) | = | 1.5 fl oz of brandy or cognac (a single jigger or shot) | = | 1.5 fl oz shot of 80-proof distilled spirits |

| about 5% alcohol | about 7% alcohol | about 12% alcohol | about 17% alcohol | about 24% alcohol | about 40% alcohol | 40% alcohol |

Fig. 1. Equivalent beverages volumes that provide the US definition of one "drink" containing 14 g of alcohol.[48]

risk for developing metabolic syndrome as well as type 2 diabetes.[39] After 24 years of follow-up, women who consumed 2 or more servings of SSBs per day had a 35% higher risk of developing coronary heart disease compared with those who consumed less than one serving/mo.[40] High fructose corn syrup (HFCS) is a common sweetener used in the beverage industry, although it is often demonized in the website and blogs. Although there are health effects associated with excessive fructose intake. HFCS does not seem to contribute any more than the direct negative health effects of those related to overall higher than recommended caloric intake.[41]

Artificial sweeteners used in beverages have become an ever more popular alternative for caloric sweeteners in SSBs, although their health effects on even basic diseases such as obesity or weight loss remain unclear, and public ability to identify them remains very poor.[42] In light of these realities, it is perhaps sensible to suggest limiting intake no more than 1 or 2 cups/d, although no soda intake is clearly preferable.

Alcohol

Moderate consumption of alcohol is generally defined as 2 drinks a day for a man or one for a woman although defining "drink equivalence" is not always simple (**Fig. 1**). Moderate alcohol consumption is protective against myocardial infarction[43] and generally not associated with increased cancer risk other than the direct link between alcohol and significantly increased risk of breast cancer in women.[44,45] Wood and colleagues (2008) observed the effect of alcohol on life expectancy in a study of 83 prospective cohort studies that included 787,000 subjects.[46] Their study concluded that for persons aged between 40 and 50 years, life expectancy was longest when alcohol intake was less than 100 g/wk or intake between 0 and 1 drink per day. Alcohol consumption in greater amounts for many, and even small amounts for some, creates many social problems, such as violence and accidents, as well as fetal alcohol syndrome when consumption occurs during pregnancy. Additionally, binge drinking and/or consistent intake of alcohol intake during pregnancy is associated with significant increased risk of miscarriage and stillbirth.[47] Moreover, of clinical note, alcohol consumption can lead to poor judgements that can lead to an inability to maintain healthy dietary recommendations (calories from alcohol consumption are rarely counted by consumers) and may adversely interact with the pharmacologic regimens that are important for those being treated for disease.

National Dietary Guidelines and Food-Related Programs

With 37 dietary components that are required for human life, it is no wonder that dietary intake, diet quality, and nutrient quantity are areas of intense research. In addition to nutrition research, several governmental and quasi-governmental organizations are responsible for setting National guidelines for dietary intake for age/sex groups including pregnancy.

Recommended dietary allowances and flour/bread enrichment—food fortification

The NAS was established by Congress in 1863. The Academy remains a key advisor to the federal government on scientific and technical matters. The NAS is a private, nonprofit, self-perpetuating society of distinguished scholars engaged in scientific and engineering research, dedicated to the furtherance of science and technology and to their use for the general welfare. The National Research Council, a division of the NAS, was charged with developing recommendations concerning the intake of the known essential nutrients for the American public. Recommended Dietary Allowances, published in 1941,[49] was developed following the start of World War Two (WWII) in Europe when it became clear that the US would require a well-nourished population and armed services. During the same time period, in 1939, the Council on Foods of the American Medical Association recommended the addition of vitamins and minerals to "general purpose foods" to restore these to the "high natural level". Two multinational companies had synthesized and were manufacturing the known vitamins and other companies had manufactured compounds of iron and calcium. Flour and bread companies were already adding different dietary components such as thiamin, B-complex, and nonfat dry milk to their products. Both the NRC and the Food and Drug Administration (FDA) agreed on the term "enriched" in 1941, and an enrichment formula was agreed to include thiamin, riboflavin, niacin, iron, vitamin D, and calcium. Thus, the First Edition of the RDA included recommendations for these 6 essential nutrients as well as for calories, protein, vitamin A, and ascorbic acid. The recommendations were for men and women at 3 different activity levels, moderately active, very active, and sedentary, pregnancy (second half), lactation, children (male and female) aged from less than 1 year to 20 years. The recommendations were for healthy people and examples of dietary patterns were included. The authors stressed that these recommendations were not standards and could change as new data became available.[49] The RDA were revised about every 5 years. The 1968 RDA formed the basis of FDA's initiative to include information about vitamin and mineral content of foods on food labels.[50] The food label, in a particularly confusing way for consumers, labeled the single value for each nutrient (that was applicable to individuals aged 4 years and older regardless of body size) as the US RDA for that nutrient.

The tenth and last edition of the RDA was published in 1989 and contained many significant changes compared with the RDA that was last published in the ninth edition.[12] The tenth edition established the RDA for vitamin K and the mineral, selenium; the RDA for folate was halved; the RDA for vitamin B12 was lowered by one-third to one-half, and the iron RDA was reduced. Because the RDAs are typically used for planning and procuring food supplies for population subgroups, including the Armed Forces and Federal prison populations, for interpreting food consumption records of individuals and populations, for establishing standards for food assistance programs, for evaluating the adequacy of food supplies in meeting national nutritional needs, for designing nutrition education programs, and for developing new products in industry, these radical changes in levels of essential nutrients were not acceptable to many nutritionists and other health professionals, and a new system was established to determine nutrient requirements. Concurrent with the publication by the NRC of the 1989 RDAs, the proceedings of a keystone meeting concerned with the role of nutrition and potential for preventing/reducing the risk of chronic diseases was published, also by the NRC.[51]

Dietary Reference Intakes (DRIs) from the National Academy of Sciences Institute of Medicine

During the next 8 years, many nutrition policy meetings were held culminating in the NAS's Institute of Medicine developing new sets of guidelines not only to prevent essential nutrient deficiencies but also to determine the potential to reduce the risk of certain chronic diseases associated with dietary intakes. The new guidelines are called Dietary Reference Intakes (DRIs). The DRIs for different sets of nutrients were published during the period 1998 to 2001. As an example, the DRI for vitamin C, vitamin E, selenium, and carotenoids was published in 2001 and has not been revised to date.[52] In 2011, revised DRIs were published only for calcium and vitamin D. None of the other DRIs has been revised since first published from 1998 to 2001.[53]

Unlike the essential nutrients, there is no universal RDA or DRI for energy (calories) because of the multitude of factors that play into an individual's energy needs. Estimation equations for energy requirements for healthy individuals are available and provide a guideline for the number of calories required to maintain a consistent weight. These equations take into account age, sex, weight, height, and level of physical activity. Available equations include infants and young children, both boys and girls aged from 3 to 8 years and from 9 to 18 years, male and female adults, and pregnant and lactating women.[54]

Food plate and the United States Department of Agriculture (USDA)

Two major food-related responsibilities of the USDA are to provide food to low-income persons and their family members and to provide guidance to Americans concerning their diet choices.

Food programs: The USDA is one of the largest Federal departments and has a myriad of programs. There are many programs that directly provide food to infants, children, and adults. USDA's domestic food and nutrition assistance programs affect the daily lives of millions of people, with about 1 in 4 Americans participating in at least one program at some point during a given year. The Supplemental Nutrition Assistance Program is the Nation's largest domestic food and nutrition assistance program for low-income Americans. The Special Supplemental Nutrition Program for WIC is the third largest USDA domestic food and nutrition assistance program. The WIC program served about 6.2 million participants per month in fiscal year 2020, including almost half of all infants born in the United States. The USDA also administers 5 other child nutrition programs: the National School Lunch Program, School Breakfast Program, Child and Adult Care Food Program, Summer Food Service Program, and After-School Snacks and Meals.

Dietary Guidelines for Americans (DGA) was first released in 1980. Since then, the DGA have become the cornerstone of Federal food and nutrition guidance.[55] The DGA provide nutritional advice for Americans who are healthy or who are at risk for chronic disease but do not currently have a chronic disease.[55] The Guidelines are published every 5 years by the USDA, together with the US Department of Health and Human Services. The purpose of the DGA is to help health professionals and policymakers to advise Americans about healthy choices for their diet. The current edition (2020–2025) is the first to include dietary guidelines for children from birth to 23 months and gives 4 overarching guidelines[56]: 1. follow a healthy dietary pattern throughout life; 2. use nutrient-dense food and beverages to reflect personal preferences, cultural traditions, and budgetary considerations; 3. meet dietary food group needs with nutrient-dense foods and beverages within calorie limits; and 4. limit foods and beverages with higher added sugars, saturated fat, and sodium, and limit alcoholic beverages. In support of these 4 guidelines, the key recommendations are as follows: avoid added sugars for infants and toddlers and limit added sugars to less than 10% of calories for those 2 years old and older; limit saturated fat to less than 10% of calories starting at age 2; limit sodium to less than 2300 mg per day (or even less if younger than 14); and limit alcoholic beverages (if consumed) to 2 drinks or less daily for men and 1 drink or less a daily for women.

The USDA initiated the use of consumer food and meal planning guidelines in 1916 and has used many pictures, including a food wheel and food guide pyramid to help consumers understand what they should consume in each meal to meet the DGA. MyPlate.gov was first developed in 2011 and was based on the 2010 version of the DGA. The current version (**Fig. 2**) is based on the current DGA, 2020 to 2025, and attempts to indicate that half of the diet (plate) should contain fruits and vegetables for each meal.[37] The 2020 to 2025 DGA advise that adults should consume 1.5 to 2 cup-equivalents of fruits and 2 to 3 cup-equivalents of vegetables daily. The latest data from the CDC indicate that in 2019, 12.3% and 10.0% of surveyed adults met fruit and vegetable intake recommendations, respectively. Meeting fruit intake recommendations was highest among Hispanic adults (16.4%) and lowest among men (10.1%). Meeting vegetable intake recommendations was highest among adults aged 51 years and older (12.5%) and lowest among adults with low income (6.8%).[57]

Nutrition Facts Label (NFL) use was mandated through the 1990 Nutrition Labeling and Education Act. The label has changed only slightly since its inception in 1994, with trans fat added to the nutrients required to be listed in 2006. In 2016, the FDA released revised rules for the NFL to help make the information on labels easier to understand for consumers and more relevant to today's nutritional needs, although some evidence argues that the new label is still confusing to the consumer.[58] Manufacturers with $10 million or more in annual sales were required to switch to the new label by January 1, 2020; manufacturers with less than $10 million in annual food sales had

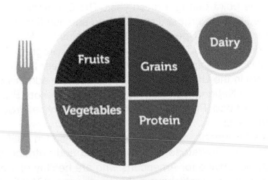

Fig. 2. Balanced nutrition education expressed with the USDA MYPLATE image.[37]

Side-by-Side Comparison

Original Label

Nutrition Facts
Serving Size 2/3 cup (55g)
Servings Per Container 8

Amount Per Serving

Calories 230   Calories from Fat 70

	% Daily Value*
Total Fat 8g	12%
Saturated Fat 1g	5%
Trans Fat 0g	
Cholesterol 0mg	0%
Sodium 160mg	7%
Total Carbohydrate 37g	12%
Dietary Fiber 4g	16%
Sugars 12g	
Protein 3g	

Vitamin A	10%
Vitamin C	8%
Calcium	20%
Iron	45%

* Percent Daily Values are based on a 2,000 calorie diet. Your Daily Value may be higher or lower depending on your calorie needs.

	Calories:	2,000	2,500
Total Fat	Less than	65g	80g
Sat Fat	Less than	20g	25g
Cholesterol	Less than	300mg	300mg
Sodium	Less than	2,400mg	2,400mg
Total Carbohydrate		300g	375g
Dietary Fiber		25g	30g

New Label

Nutrition Facts
8 servings per container
Serving size   2/3 cup (55g)

Amount per serving
Calories   230

	% Daily Value*
Total Fat 8g	10%
Saturated Fat 1g	5%
Trans Fat 0g	
Cholesterol 0mg	0%
Sodium 160mg	7%
Total Carbohydrate 37g	13%
Dietary Fiber 4g	14%
Total Sugars 12g	
Includes 10g Added Sugars	**20%**
Protein 3g	

Vitamin D 2mcg	10%
Calcium 260mg	20%
Iron 8mg	45%
Potassium 240mg	6%

* The % Daily Value (DV) tells you how much a nutrient in a serving of food contributes to a daily diet. 2,000 calories a day is used for general nutrition advice.

Fig. 3. Comparison of new and old nutrition facts labels used for consumer nutrition education.[59]

until January 1, 2021 to comply.[59] Thus, the current, more complex label is a recent advancement for providing consumers more information on food labels (**Fig. 3.**)[59]

CDC monitors the health of the US population and at the same time, surveys the nutritional status of the population. The National Center for Health Statistics, which is under the CDC has been looking at the health and nutritional status of the US population since the 1960s. NHANES II 1976–1980, provided by the National Center for Health Statistics, is a program of studies designed to assess the health and nutritional status of adults and children in the United States. The survey is unique in that it combines interviews and physical examinations. In 1999, the survey became a continuous program that has a changing focus on a variety of health and nutrition measurements to meet emerging needs. The survey examines a nationally representative sample of about 5000 persons each year. These persons are located in counties across the country, 15 of which are visited each year. The data from the NHANES surveys provide the major documentation for the development of the US dietary recommendations and guidelines.[60]

Nutritional Challenges of the Evolving COVID-19 Pandemic

Food insecurity occurs when people lack consistent access to enough food for a normal active life. It was previously considered that basic nutrition has changed during these first 2 years of the COVID-19 pandemic. COVID-19 lockdowns, quarantine, and changing food delivery systems have changed food intake, eating behaviors, and dietary quality in Europe and most countries.[61] The lockdown has generally increased the tendency to cook at home and has been associated with increased fruit, vegetable, legume, and water intake, with decreased red meat intake, what most clinicians would call "dietary improvement." However, these average improvements are balanced by tremendous COVID-19-related increases in food insecurity and malnutrition experienced by those who are elderly, schoolchildren no longer coming to schools, unemployed, clinically depressed, and those in disadvantaged socioeconomic status.[62] It is well known that malnutrition is a risk factor for many diseases, and COVID-19 is no different.

COVID-19 has fundamentally changed the basic food delivery systems that determine access to our diet and the status of our resulting nutritional quality. Lockdowns and quarantines made access to raw or processed foods more complicated and potentially unsafe even for those with prior vaccination.[63] Deliveries of retail grocery products through online orders can be made through Amazon, Walmart, and a variety of delivery apps and intermediary facilitators. Premade restaurant items can be delivered through Grubhub, DoorDash, Uber Eats, and a plethora of other intermediaries. Home meal kits that provide all components for prepare-at-home meals for an entire week or more can be sent in a box through the mail can through companies such as Freshly.com. However, these functionaries require economic resources, online or Wifi access, a credit card for making purchases, and online literacy. The elderly, racial minorities, single parents, and those with physical or mental handicaps including those who may not have access to food delivery resources are at greater risk of food insecurity and malnutrition,[64] which is associated with increases the risk and severity of COVID-19 infection.

Nutritional needs change further when a person is infected but not hospitalized with COVID-19 because the ability to feed ones-self or access food while at home under quarantine may be impaired. In recent US study of 192,550 adults who were hospitalized for COVID-19, the duration of the COVID-19 stay for non-Intensive Care Unit (ICU) patients was 6 days and 15 days with ICU admittance with nutrition-related comorbidities at admittance including hypertension (61.5%), diabetes (38.4%), and obesity (27.4%).[65] COVID-19 mechanical ventilation was typically required for 15 days (1–85 days range) and total hospital stay before discharge was 25 days (7–86 days range). Mechanical ventilation recipients require either enteral or parenteral nutrition that requires very specialized nutritional attention that is further complicated by the aforementioned COVID-19 comorbidities.[66]

Direct COVID-19 infection, quarantine due to contact with infected family members, or fear related to COVID-19 risk factors have led to unprecedented labor shortages and inability to monitor patient nutrition when patient monitoring needs are greatest.[67]

Clinical ability to tailor nutritional demands for those with hypertension, diabetes, and obesity would otherwise be paramount during an ICU stay. During longer periods of inactivity related to lockdown or hospitalization, the elderly and those on ventilators are at great risk of significant muscle wasting and sarcopenia.[68] These nutritional complications are experienced at the exact time when access to intensive dietary therapy is hindered by COVID-19-dependent work force reductions and patient hospitalization overload.

Specific nutrient interactions may predict either severity of disease or the potential for protection from the clinical manifestations of COVID-19. Vitamin D is readily synthesized when the skin is exposed to direct sunlight especially during summer months; however, stay-at-home and other lockdown protocols can result in deficiencies. In this regard, low vitamin D levels have been shown to be highly correlated with increased COVID-19 infection rates and symptom severity.[69] Moreover, dietary supplementation studies, such as those using zinc[70] show promise as does a simple recommendation that the population seek more direct sunlight to enhance vitamin D synthesis. Because the COVID-19 cytokine storm induces a proinflammatory response, a great interest has developed in vitamins such as vitamin D, minerals such as zinc, and antioxidants such as vitamin C and glutathione for a potential role as part of COVID-19 prevention, treatment, and recovery,[71] although definitive randomized intervention studies for the utility of these supplements have been negative, to date.

SUMMARY

Approximately 80% of the major chronic diseases, such as obesity, diabetes, hypertension, and diet-related cancers, are at least partly preventable with better nutrition. Unfortunately, medical training and practice is focused on the treatment of these conditions after their diagnosis. It is critically important that both the clinician and the patient understand that humans are required to consume a varied diet that contains sufficient liquids and the essential vitamins, mineral, fats, and amino acids necessary for life. General fluency with respect to the health effects of water, tea, coffee, SSBs is also an area of intense patient interest and clinical significance. An improved understanding of the governmental organizations responsible for nutrition recommendations and the use of NFLs on food products can improve health outcomes. Growth charts, BMI, and caloric need calculations are also important clinical nutrition considerations. Finally, the complications to food availability, delivery, and nutrition assessment in relation to the ongoing COVID pandemic will continue to stress our ability to provide the most data-driven recommendations concerning nutrition for health, disease prevention, and treatment. It is clear that much needs to be done to avoid a continuation of the increase in deaths associated with many different diet-based preventable conditions. It is true that the scientific basis of nutrition recommendations is constantly changing, as is true for all science/research-based fields. This article can help the clinician understand the changes that have led to the current diet recommendations and can remind the patient that as more nutrition research is done, the recommendations will further improve their nutrition and overall health.

CLINICS CARE POINTS

- Both the clinician and the patient understand that humans are required to consume a varied diet that contains sufficient liquids and the essential vitamins, mineral, fats, and amino acids necessary for life.

- Growth charts, BMI, and caloric need calculations are also important clinical nutrition.considerations.
- The complications to food availability, delivery, and nutrition assessment in relation to the ongoing COVID pandemic will continue to stress our ability to provide the most data-driven recommendations concerning nutrition for health, disease prevention, and treatment.

DISCLOSURE

Drs T. Wilson and A. Bendich have no disclosures.

REFERENCES

1. Micha R, Peñalvo JL, Cudhea F, et al. Association between dietary factors and mortality from heart disease, stroke, and type 2 diabetes in the United States. JAMA 2017;317:912–24.
2. Catov JM, Bodnar LM, Olsen J, et al. Periconceptional multivitamin use and risk of preterm or small-for-gestational-age births in the Danish National Birth Cohort. Am J Clin Nutr 2011;94:906–12.
3. Czeizel AE, Vereczkey A, Szabó I. Folic acid in pregnant women associated with reduced prevalence of severe congenital heart defects in their children: a national population-based case-control study. Eur J Obstet Gynecol Reprod Biol 2015;193:34–9.
4. Adams KM, Kohlmeier M, Zeisel SH. Nutrition education in U.S. medical schools: latest update of a national survey. Acad Med 2010;85:1537–42.
5. Devries S, Willett W, Bonow RO. Nutrition education in medical school, residency training, and practice. JAMA 2019;321:1351–2.
6. Olsen JA, Vitamin A. Handbook of vitamins. In: Machlin LJ, editor. 2nd Edition. New York: Marcel Dekker; 1991. p. 2–57.
7. Moser U, Bendich A. Vitamin C In: Handbook of vitamins. In: Machlin LJ, editor. 2nd Edition. New York; 1991. p. 196–232.
8. Vitamin intake and health, edited by Gaby S.K, Bendich A., Singh V. N., et al, 1991, pp 1-16.
9. Stephenson T, Sanctuary MR, Passerrello CW. Human nutrition: science for healthy living. New York City, New York: McGraw-Hill; 2022.
10. Chromium. In: Dietary reference intakes for vitamin A, vitamin K, arsenic, boron, chromium, iodine, iron, manganese, molybdenum, nickel, silicon, vanadium, and chromium. Institute of medicine (US) panel on micronutrients. Washington (DC): National Academies Press; 2001. p. 197–223.
11. Lands, W.E.M. Polyunsaturated fatty acid effects on cellular interactions. In: Micronutrients in health and in disease prevention, edited by Bendich A and Butterworth C E, New York: 1991, pp 9-34.
12. National Research Council. Recommended dietary allowances. 10th edition. Washington (DC): The National Academies Press; 1989. https://doi.org/10.17226/1349.
13. Rose WC, Haines WJ, Warner DT. The amino acid requirements of man. III. The role of isoleucine; additional evidence concerning histidine. J Biol Chem 2016; 193:605–12.
14. Dinicolantonio JJ. Increase in the intake of refined carbohydrates and sugar may have led to the health decline of the Greenland Eskimos. Open Heart 2016;3(2): e000444.

15. Statistics Canada. Health reports. modified 2015 82-003-x 19(1). Available at: https://www150.statcan.gc.ca/n1/pub/82-003-x/2008001/article/10463/4149059-eng.htm. Accessed January 10, 2022.
16. Schulz R, Slavin J. Perspective: defining carbohydrate quality for human health and environmental sustainability. Adv Nutr 2021;12:1108–21.
17. National Center for Health Statistics. Growth charts. centers for disease control and prevention. Available at. https://www.cdc.gov/growthcharts/. Accessed February 22, 2022.
18. Romero-Corral A, Somers VK, Sierra-Johnson J, et al. Accuracy of body mass index in diagnosing obesity in the adult general population. Int J Obes (Lond) 2008;32:959–66.
19. Barry VW, Baruth M, Beets MW, et al. Fitness vs. fatness on all-cause mortality: a meta-analysis. Prog Cardiovasc Dis 2014;56(4):382–90.
20. National Academies of Sciences, Engineering, and Medicine. Dietary reference intakes for water, potassium, sodium, chloride, and sulfate. Washington (DC): The National Academies Press; 2005. https://doi.org/10.17226/10925.
21. Vivanti AP. Origins for the estimations of water requirements in adults. Eur J Clin Nutr 2012;66:1282–9.
22. Bellinger DC. Lead contamination in flint–an abject failure to protect public health. N Engl J Med 2016;374:1101–3.
23. Carlson JR, Bauer BA, Vincent A, et al. Reading the tea leaves: anticarcinogenic properties of (-)-epigallocatechin-3-gallate. Mayo Clin Proc 2007;82:725–32.
24. Basu A, Lucas EA. Mechanisms and effects of green tea on cardiovascular health. Nutr Rev 2007;65:361–75.
25. Wang ZM, Zhou B, Wang YS, et al. Black and green tea consumption and the risk of coronary artery disease: a meta-analysis. Am J Clin Nutr 2011;93:506–15.
26. Teramoto M, Muraki I, Yamagishi K, et al. Green tea and coffee consumption and all-cause mortality among persons with and without stroke or myocardial infarction. Stroke 2021;52:957–65.
27. Miranda AM, Goulart AC, Benseñor IM, et al. Coffee consumption and risk of hypertension: a prospective analysis in the cohort study. Clin Nutr 2021;40:542–9.
28. Ding M, Bhupathiraju SN, Satija A, et al. Long-term coffee consumption and risk of cardiovascular disease: a systematic review and a dose-response meta-analysis of prospective cohort studies. Circulation 2014;129:643–59.
29. Santos RM, Lima DR. Coffee consumption, obesity and type 2 diabetes: a mini-review. Eur J Nutr 2016;55:1345–58.
30. Dong X, Li S, Sun J, et al. Association of coffee, decaffeinated coffee and caffeine intake from coffee with cognitive performance in older adults: national health and nutrition examination survey (NHANES) 2011-2014. Nutrients 2020;12:840.
31. Alicandro G, Tavani A, La Vecchia C. Coffee and cancer risk: a summary overview. Eur J Cancer Prev 2017;26:424–32.
32. Appel LJ, Moore TJ, Obarzanek E, et al. A clinical trial of the effects of dietary patterns on blood pressure. N Engl J Med 1997;336:1117–24.
33. Soedamah-Muthu SS, Ding EL, Al-Delaimy WK, et al. Milk and dairy consumption and incidence of cardiovascular diseases and all-cause mortality: dose-response meta-analysis of prospective cohort studies. Am J Clin Nutr 2011;93: 158–71.
34. Good Food Institute. U.S. Retail market data for the plant-based industry. Available at. https://gfi.org/marketresearch/#:~:text=Plant%2Dbased%20milk%20is%20the,%2C%20growing%2045%25%20since%202019. Accessed: January 18, 2022.

35. Craig WJ, Brothers CJ, Mangels R. Nutritional content and health profile of single-serve non-dairy plant-based beverages. Nutrients 2021;14162.
36. Collard KM, McCormick DP. A nutritional comparison of cow's milk and alternative milk products. Acad Pediatr 2021;21:1067–9.
37. MyPlate. US. Department of Agriculture. Available at: https://www.myplate.gov/eat-healthy/fruits.
38. Popkin BM. Patterns of beverage use across the lifecycle. Physiol Behav 2010; 100:4–9.
39. Malik VS, Popkin BM, Bray GA, et al. Sugar-sweetened beverages and risk of metabolic syndrome and type 2 diabetes: a meta-analysis. Diabetes Care 2010;33:2477–83.
40. Fung TT, Malik V, Rexrode KM, et al. Sweetened beverage consumption and risk of coronary heart disease in women. Am J Clin Nutr 2009;89:1037–42.
41. Zafar MI, Frese M, Mills KE. Chronic fructose substitution for glucose or sucrose in food or beverages and metabolic outcomes: an updated systematic review and meta-analysis. Front Nutr 2021;8:647600.
42. Wilson T, Murray B, Price T, et al. Non-nutritive (Artificial) sweetener knowledge among university students. Nutrients 2019;11:E2201.
43. Mukamal KJ, Jensen MK, Grønbaek M, et al. Drinking frequency, mediating biomarkers, and risk of myocardial infarction in women and men. Circulation 2005; 112:1406–13.
44. Cao Y, Willett WC, Rimm EB, et al. Light to moderate intake of alcohol, drinking patterns, and risk of cancer: results from two prospective US cohort studies. BMJ 2015;18:351, h4238.
45. Willett WC. Public health benefits of preventive nutrition: global perspective. In: Bendich A, Deckelbaum RJ, editors. Preventive nutrition. 5th edition. New York: Humana Press, Springer/Nature; 2015. p. 25–46.
46. Wood AM, Kaptoge S, Butterworth AS, et al. Risk thresholds for alcohol consumption: combined analysis of individual-participant data for 599 912 current drinkers in 83 prospective studies. Lancet 2018;391:1513–23.
47. Gosdin LK, Deputy NP, Kim SY, et al. Alcohol consumption and binge drinking during pregnancy among adults aged 18–49 years — United States, 2018–2020. MMWR Morb Mortal Wkly Rep 2022;71:10–3.
48. National Institute of Standards and Technology. How do you know your food's nutrition label is accurate? National Institute on Alcohol Abuse and Alcoholism. National Institutes of Health. US Department of Health and Human Services. Rethinking Drinking. Available at: http://rethinkingdrinking.niaaa.nih.gov/How-much-is-too-much/What-counts-as-a-drink/Whats-A-Standard-Drink.aspx. Accessed: January 7, 2022.
49. National Research Council. Recommended dietary allowances. Washington (DC): The National Academies Press; 1941. https://doi.org/10.17226/13286. Available at:.
50. National Research Council (U.S). Food and nutrition board. Recommended dietary allowances; a report of the food and nutrition board. Washington (DC): National Academy of Sciences-National Research Council; 1968.
51. National Research Council. Diet and health: implications for reducing chronic disease risk. Report of the committee on diet and health, food and nutrition board, commission on life sciences. Washington (DC): National Academies Press; 1989. p. 750.
52. Dietary reference intakes (DRIS): recommended intakes for individuals, food and nutrition board, institute of medicine. National Academies; 2004.

53. The development of DRIS 1994-2004: lessons learned and new challenges: workshop summary. institute of medicine. Washington (DC): The National Academies Press; 2008. https://doi.org/10.17226/12086. Available at:.

54. Mifflin MD, St Jeor ST, Hill LA, et al. A new predictive equation for resting energy expenditure in healthy individuals. Am J Clin Nutr 1990;51:241–7.

55. United States Department of Agriculture. United States department of health and human services nutrition and your health: dietary guidelines for Americans. Washington (DC): Government Printing Office; 1980.

56. United States Department of Health and Human Services, United States Department of Agriculture Dietary Guidelines for Americans, 2015–2020. Washington (DC): United States Department of Health and Human Services and United States Department of Agriculture; 2015. Contract No.: HHS-ODPHP-2015-2020-01-DGA-A Home and Garden Bulletin No. 232.

57. Lee SH, Moore LV, Park S, et al. Adults meeting fruit and vegetable intake recommendations-united states, 2019. MMWR Morb Mortal Wkly Rep 2022; 71:1–9.

58. Kim EJ, Ellison B, Prescott MP, et al. Consumer comprehension of the nutrition facts label: a comparison of the original and updated labels. Am J Health Promot 2021;35:648–57.

59. U.S. DEPARTMENT OF AGRICULTURE. Food labeling. economic research service. Available at: https://www.ers.usda.gov/topics/food-choices-health/consumer-information-and-labeling/food-labeling/#labels. Accessed February 23, 2022.

60. Center for Disease Control. About the national health and nutrition examination survey. Available at: https://www.cdc.gov/nchs/nhanes/about_nhanes.htm. Accessed January 19, 2022.

61. Mignogna C, Costanzo S, Ghulam A, et al. Impact of nationwide lockdowns resulting from the first wave of the COVID-19 pandemic on food intake, eating behaviours and diet quality: a systematic review. Adv Nutr 2021;nmab130.

62. Choi SL, Men F. Food insecurity associated with higher COVID-19 infection in households with older adults. Public Health 2021;200:7–14.

63. Dana LM, Hart E, mcaleese A, et al. Factors associated with ordering food via online meal ordering services. Public Health Nutr 2021;24:5704–9.

64. Keeble M, Adams J, Bishop TRP, et al. Socioeconomic inequalities in food outlet access through an online food delivery service in England: A cross-sectional descriptive analysis. Appl Geogr 2021;133:102498, j.apgeog.2021.

65. Nguyen NT, Chinn J, Nahmias J, et al. Outcomes and mortality among adults hospitalized with COVID-19 at US medical centers. JAMA Netw Open 2021;4: e210417.

66. Thibault R, Seguin P, Tamion F, et al. Nutrition of the COVID-19 patient in the intensive care unit (ICU): a practical guidance. Crit Care 2020;24:447.

67. Defense department will help relieve 2 Minnesota hospitals. Available at: https://www.mprnews.org/story/2021/11/17/defense-department-will-help-relieve-2-minnesota-hospitals. Accessed January 6, 2022.

68. Wierdsma NJ, Kruizenga HM, Konings LA, et al. Poor nutritional status, risk of sarcopenia and nutrition related complaints are prevalent in COVID-19 patients during and after hospital admission. Clin Nutr ESPEN 2021;43:369–76.

69. Yisak H, Ewunetei A, Kefale B, et al. Effects of vitamin D on COVID-19 infection and prognosis: a systematic review. Risk Manag Healthc Policy 2021;14:31–8.

70. Cereda G, Ciappolino V, Boscutti A, et al. Zinc as a neuroprotective nutrient for COVID-19-related neuropsychiatric manifestations: a literature review. Adv Nutr 2021;11:nmab110.

71. Fiorino S, Gallo C, Zippi M, et al. Cytokine storm in aged people with cov-2: possible role of vitamins as therapy or preventive strategy. Aging Clin Exp Res 2020;32:2115–31.

Medical and Surgical Treatment of Obesity

Tirissa J. Reid, MD[a,b,]*, Judith Korner, MD, PhD[a,c]

KEYWORDS

- Overweight • Obesity • Medication • Pharmacotherapy • Medical devices
- Endoscopic therapies • Bariatric surgery

KEY POINTS

- Antiobesity medications and devices should be considered for patients with a body mass index (BMI) $\geq$ 30 kg/m^2 or a BMI 27 to 30 kg/m^2 with weight-related comorbidities if unable to lose or maintain weight loss using lifestyle interventions.
- Antiobesity devices and endoscopic therapies should be considered for patients with a BMI $\geq$ 25 to 55 kg/m^2, depending on the device
- Bariatric surgery should be considered for patients with a BMI $\geq$ 40 kg/m^2 or a BMI $\geq$ 35 kg/m^2 with weight-related comorbidities.
- Antiobesity medications, devices, and bariatric surgery should always be used in conjunction with a lifestyle intervention.

INTRODUCTION

The prevalence rate for obesity in the United States has continued to rise steadily since the 1980s and is most recently at 42.4% in adults.[1] During this time period, few effective therapies have been developed for obesity. During this same time, the creation of therapies for other conditions, such as hypertension, has blossomed to more than 70 antihypertensive medications.[2] There are currently five Food and Drug Administration (FDA)-approved medications, several medical devices and bariatric surgery options for chronic therapy of obesity yet training in the management of obesity remains minimal in medical school and residency programs.[3–7] This leaves many medical residents feeling unequipped to manage patients with obesity once they move into clinical practice.[4,5] This chapter provides an overview of medical

[a] Division of Endocrinology, Diabetes & Metabolism, Department of Medicine, Vagelos College of Physicians and Surgeons, Columbia University Irving Medical Center, New York, NY, USA; [b] Vagelos College of Physicians and Surgeons, Columbia University Irving Medical Center, 161 Fort Washington Avenue, Room 512, New York, NY 10032, USA; [c] Vagelos College of Physicians and Surgeons, Columbia University Irving Medical Center, 650 West 168th Street, Black Building, Room 20-08, New York, NY 10032, USA
* Corresponding author. Vagelos College of Physicians and Surgeons, Columbia University Irving Medical Center, 161 Fort Washington Avenue, Room 512, New York, NY 10032.
E-mail address: tjr2122@cumc.columbia.edu

Med Clin N Am 106 (2022) 837–852
https://doi.org/10.1016/j.mcna.2022.03.002
0025-7125/22/© 2022 Elsevier Inc. All rights reserved.
medical.theclinics.com

therapies to assist primary care providers in the management of patients with obesity and to guide the choice of the appropriate medical treatment modality.

BACKGROUND

Two percent of patients who are eligible for antiobesity medications receive a prescription for this therapy.[8-11] Less than 1% of patients who are eligible for bariatric surgery undergo surgery.[12-14] Reasons for such limited use of these modalities are many, including an incomplete understanding of the pathogenesis of obesity, unfamiliarity with the risk–benefit profile of available medical and surgical treatments, as well as hesitancy in using antiobesity medications due to a history of some prior medication recalls.[11,13,15-17] In 2013, the American Medical Association recognized that obesity is a disease.[18] This disease is characterized by metabolic dysfunction involving multiple organ systems, including the gut, brain, muscle, and adipose tissue. A diagnosis of obesity increases the risk for more than 50 diseases with significant morbidity and mortality.[19] Multiple studies have shown that a modest sustained weight loss of 5%–10% or greater can have a positive impact on many weight-related comorbidities, including type 2 diabetes mellitus (T2DM), hypertension, obstructive sleep apnea, nonalcoholic fatty liver disease, osteoarthritis, polycystic ovarian syndrome, infertility, and idiopathic intracranial hypertension.[20-23]

DEFINITIONS

Overweight = body mass index (BMI) 25–29.9 kg/m^2
  Obesity = BMI $\geq$ 30 kg/m^2
  BMI = weight (in kg)/height (m^2)

EVALUATION

Before considering antiobesity pharmacotherapy, a thorough weight-focused history and physical exam, including BMI, should be performed. The evaluation should include information about the patient's trajectory of weight gain, prior weight loss attempts, including lifestyle interventions, pharmacotherapy, and bariatric surgery and their results. The review of systems and physical exam should be evaluated with an eye to detect any undiagnosed weight-related comorbidities and medical conditions, which can result in weight gain or make weight loss more difficult. This would include hypothyroidism, obstructive sleep apnea, polycystic ovarian syndrome, hypogonadism, or the less common Cushing's disease. Special attention should be paid to the patient's chronic medications to determine whether medications that promote weight gain may be switched to an equally effective medication that is weight neutral or promotes weight loss.[24] Frequently prescribed medication classes that promote weight gain include beta-blockers for hypertension, antipsychotics, antidepressants, antiepileptics, and antihyperglycemic medications. For instance, insulin and sulfonylureas for the treatment of T2DM cause weight gain and in some cases may be substituted with weight neutral medications such as dipeptidyl peptidase-4 (DPP-4) inhibitors or metformin, sodium-glucose cotransporter 2 (SGLT-2) inhibitors, and glucagon-like peptide-1 (GLP-1) receptor agonists that promote weight loss.

APPROACH

Patients with a BMI $\geq$ 30 kg/m^2 or BMI 27 to 29.9 kg/m^2 with a weight-related comorbidity who have not been successful at losing and/or maintaining at least 5% of their weight after 6 months of a comprehensive lifestyle intervention are candidates for antiobesity pharmacotherapy. The World Health Organization suggests lower BMI criteria be used in Asian populations to determine overweight and obesity for whom a BMI 23–27.5 kg/m^2 is overweight and 27.5 kg/m^2 or higher is obesity.[25] This recommendation is due to studies showing that weight-related comorbidities develop at lower BMIs in Asian populations. After eligibility for medication therapy has been established, a patient's readiness to participate in a weight-loss intervention should be assessed.[26]

GUIDELINES

American Heart Association/American College of Cardiology/The Obesity Society Guidelines contain an algorithm to guide providers on when to institute lifestyle changes, antiobesity pharmacotherapy and/or bariatric surgery.[24,26] It is important to keep in mind that an intensive lifestyle intervention is the initial therapy for any patient who has not previously attempted weight loss. Lifestyle changes should remain the backbone of therapy, even if escalated to pharmacotherapy, a medical device, or bariatric surgery.

THERAPEUTIC OPTIONS
Pharmacotherapy

There is currently one class of medications that are FDA approved for short-term antiobesity therapy and five medications that are FDA approved for chronic therapy, recognizing that obesity is a chronic disease.

There is no way to predict which medication will be most effective for any given patient as responses to medication therapy follow a bell-shaped curve, with wide interindividual variability. The initial choice of therapy should be based on whether a patient has a comorbid condition that can be treated, along with whether patients have contraindications to specific medications. As with all other medications, patients should be monitored closely for response and the medication should be changed if a patient has adverse effects or the medication is not effective for them. Endocrine Society Clinical Practice guidelines recommend that patients be monitored at least monthly for the initial 3 months on pharmacotherapy and then at least every 3–6 months thereafter.[24] Regardless of which medication is used, it is important to remember that concurrent lifestyle changes are key to achieving optimal results. **Table 1** details the current FDA-approved medications for treating obesity, which are briefly described below, including their mechanism of action, dosing, mean weight loss, contraindications, and common adverse effects.[27]

Sympathomimetic agents, such as phentermine and diethylpropion, were approved by the FDA approximately 60 years ago for short-term obesity therapy of 3 months' duration. They cause weight loss through a decrease in appetite and an increase in metabolism. Mean weight loss is 2–10 kg greater than placebo at 3 months.[28]

Phentermine/topiramate-extended release was FDA approved for therapy of obesity in July 2012. This medication is a combination of phentermine, described above, with topiramate, which is FDA approved as monotherapy for epilepsy and migraine headaches. At 1 year, subjects on the 15/92 mg dose had a 10.9% total body weight loss (TBWL) versus 1.6% TBWL in the placebo group; 66.7% of subjects on the 15/92 mg dose experienced ≥5% TBWL, which is the criteria for efficacy with antiobesity medications.[29] The risk for progression to T2DM was decreased by 76% in the 15/92 mg group over 4 years.[30]

Orlistat 120 mg was FDA approved in 1999, and a lower 60 mg nonprescription formulation was FDA approved in 2007. Orlistat is a pancreatic lipase inhibitor that

Table 1
Antiobesity pharmacotherapy

Medication	Dose	Mean % Total Body Weight Loss (Time)	Contraindications	Adverse Effects
Sympathomimetic agents: Phentermine Diethylpropion	Phentermine: 8 mg, 15 mg, 30 mg, 37.5 mg po daily Diethylpropion: 120 mg po tid	2–10 kg (3 mo)	• CVD • Uncontrolled HTN • Severe anxiety • Seizure disorder • MAOI use	• Dry mouth • Increased heart rate or BP • Headache • Insomnia • Irritability • Constipation • Diarrhea
Orlistat	60 mg OTC or 120 mg po tid qac	8.8% at 1 y (120 mg)	• Malabsorptive syndrome	• Abdominal bloating • Flatulence • Diarrhea • Malabsorption of fat-soluble vitamins (ADEK)
Phentermine-topiramate CR	3.75–23 mg po daily x 2 wk, then 7.5–46 mg po daily (if insufficient weight loss may titrate up): 11.25–69 mg po daily x 2 wk, 15–92 mg po daily	10.9% at 1 y (15–92 mg)	• CVD • Uncontrolled HTN • Glaucoma • Risk of pregnancy (teratogen: incr risk for cleft lip/palate)	• Dry mouth • Increased heart rate or BP • Insomnia • Irritability • Constipation • Paresthesias • Fatigue • Decreased concentration/memory • Nephrolithiasis
Naltrexone SR 8 mg-Bupropion SR 90 mg	Titrate up every week from 1 tab po daily to 2 tabs po bid	6.1% at 1 y	• Uncontrolled HTN • Seizure disorder • Chronic opioid use • History of bulimia • MAOI use	• Nausea • Vomiting • Constipation • Headache • Dizziness • Insomnia

| Liraglutide | Titrate up every week from 0.6 mg SC daily to 1.2 mg, 1.8 mg, 2.4 mg, 3 mg SC daily | 8.0% at 1 y | • Personal or family history of medullary thyroid cancer or MEN2 syndrome | • Nausea
• Vomiting
• Diarrhea
• Constipation
• GERD
Rare:
• Pancreatitis
• Cholelithiasis |
| Semaglutide | Titrate up every 4 wk from 0.25 mg SC once a week to 0.5 mg, 1.0 mg, 1.7 mg, 2.4 mg SC once a week | 16.0% at 68 wk | • Personal or family history of medullary thyroid cancer or MEN2 syndrome | • Same as liraglutide |

blocks the absorption of 30% of ingested fat. At 1 year, subjects on orlistat 120 mg had 8.8% TBWL versus 5.8% TBWL in the placebo group; 65.7% and 38.9% on orlistat 120 mg experienced ≥5% and ≥10% TBWL, respectively. Low-density lipoprotein cholesterol showed a significant decrease of 8 mg/dL at 2 years compared with the placebo group.[31]

Naltrexone HCl/bupropion HCl extended release combines naltrexone, FDA approved as monotherapy for alcohol and opioid abuse, with bupropion, FDA approved as monotherapy for depression and smoking cessation. This combination was FDA approved in 2014 and works centrally to increase the activity of anorexigenic proopiomelanocortin (POMC) neurons in the hypothalamus and central nervous system reward pathways to decrease appetite and increase energy expenditure.[32,33] Mean weight loss on naltrexone/bupropion at 1 year was 6.1% TBWL versus 1.3% TBWL on placebo; 48% and 25% experienced ≥5% and ≥10% TBWL, respectively.[34,35]

Liraglutide, FDA approved for obesity therapy in December 2014, is a subcutaneous daily injection in the medication class of glucagon-like peptide-1 receptor (GLP-1R) agonists. These agonists act on the central nervous system to decrease appetite and slow gastric emptying to increase satiety. At 1 year, subjects achieved an 8.0% TBWL versus 2.6% in the placebo group, with 63.2% losing ≥5% TBWL and 33.1% losing ≥10% TBWL.[36] More than 2 years, it reduced the prevalence of prediabetes in study subjects by greater than 50%.[37] This class of medication is FDA approved to treat T2DM, which it does primarily by increasing postprandial insulin secretion. Of note, major cardiovascular events were significantly reduced in patients with T2DM treated with liraglutide compared with placebo.[38]

Semaglutide is a subcutaneous weekly GLP-1R agonist, which was approved for obesity therapy in June 2021. This medication was previously approved at a lower dose for the treatment of T2DM. At the higher dose of 2.4 mg, it has greater effects on appetite and satiety, resulting in a mean of 16.0% TBWL versus 5.7% TBWL on placebo after 68 weeks; 75.3% of patients achieved ≥10% TBWL and 55.8% ≥ 15% TBWL at 68 weeks.[39,40] A phase 2 trial involving patients with nonalcoholic steatohepatitis (NASH) showed that treatment with semaglutide resulted in a significantly higher percentage of patients with NASH resolution than placebo.[41]

Metformin is FDA approved for the treatment of T2DM but is frequently used off-label for prediabetes, polycystic ovary syndrome, and to assist with weight loss. This treatment is based on the Diabetes Prevention Program trial, which demonstrated that metformin promotes a modest weight loss and decreases the risk of progression to diabetes by 31% over 4 years in patients who had a BMI of ≥ 24 kg/m², a fasting glucose between 95 and 125 mg/dL and an elevated oral glucose tolerance test value between 140 and 199 mg/dL at 2 h after a 75 g oral glucose load.[42]

Medical Devices/Endoscopic Therapies

Table 2 lists antiobesity medical devices and endoscopic therapies, mode of administration or placement, mean weight loss, contraindications and adverse events.

Cellulose hydrogel capsules were FDA approved in June 2019 for patients with a BMI of ≥ 25–40 kg/m². These capsules are ingested with water before lunch and dinner and the superabsorbent particles absorb water to form a three-dimensional matrix, which occupies 25% of stomach volume, increasing satiety and decreasing the amount of food ingested. Although contained in capsules, this is considered a medical device as it is not systemically absorbed, and its mechanism of action is mechanical. At 6 months, mean TBWL was 6.4% in the active treatment group versus 4.3% in the placebo group; 59% achieved ≥ 5% TBWL and 27.2% achieved ≥ 10% TBWL. Of

Table 2
Antiobesity medical devices and endoscopic therapies

Name	Administration/ Placement	Mean % Total Body Weight Loss (Time)	Contraindications	Adverse Events
Cellulose hydrogel	3 caps po tid qac	6.4% (6 mo)	• History of prior GI surgery	• Diarrhea Rare: • Bowel obstruction
Intragastric Balloons	Placed via endoscopy or swallowable capsule	12%–14% (6 mo)	• History of prior GI surgery	• Nausea • Vomiting • Heartburn • Diarrhea • Abdominal discomfort Rare: • Bowel obstruction • Perforation
Gastric Aspiration Device	Placed similar to gastrostomy tube	12.1% (1 y)	• History of bulimia or binge eating disorder • Prior gastric surgery	• Indigestion • Nausea • Vomiting • Periostomal infection

note, the greatest mean %TBWL was seen in patients with prediabetes and treatment-naïve diabetes. These patients had a mean of 8.1% TBWL and were six times more likely to achieve ≥ 10% TBWL at 6 months, noted in 44% of this subgroup.[43]

Intragastric balloons are FDA approved to treat patients with a BMI of 30–40 kg/m^2. They are inserted via endoscopy or by swallowing a capsule, remain in place for 6 months, and occupy space to increase satiety and decrease the amount of food ingested, resulting in a mean of 12%–14.4% TBWL at 6 months. Removal is performed using endoscopy. Close follow-up and adherence to lifestyle changes are required to maintain weight loss after removal. Studies show a regain of 28%–36% of the weight lost 1 year after removal.[44–46]

The gastric aspiration device is an endoscopically placed gastrostomy tube through which fluid is infused postmeal, with an external device for drainage. It is FDA approved for patients with a BMI of 35–55 kg/m^2. In a 10-min process, 30% of gastric contents are aspirated postmeal, decreasing caloric absorption and resulting in weight loss. Mean %TBWL is 12.1% at 1 year with the device versus 3.5% TBWL in a lifestyle intervention group.[47]

Bariatric Surgery

The bariatric surgeries discussed are listed in **Table 3**, along with their mean weight loss and adverse events.[48,49]

Laparoscopic adjustable gastric banding (LAGB) involves the placement of a hollow, circular band with an inner inflatable balloon near the top of the stomach, which is connected to a port in the abdomen. Saline is inserted into the port to inflate the balloon and restrict the amount of food that can be ingested, resulting in a mean of 13.7% TBWL at 1 year and 11.7% TBWL at 5 years.[48] This is currently the least performed bariatric surgery due to lack of durable weight loss and complications such as band slippage or gastric erosion, requiring removal.

Sleeve gastrectomy (SG) involves the removal of approximately 80% of the stomach, and the remaining portion of the stomach resembles the shape of a tube. The smaller stomach restricts the amount of food ingested and results in a mean of 25.2% TBWL at 1 year and 18.8% TBWL at 5 years.[48]

Roux-en-Y gastric bypass (RYGB) involves the division of the stomach to create a smaller gastric pouch for food and attachment of the jejunum to the new gastric pouch. Ingested food bypasses the duodenum and proximal jejunum, which are usually the main sites of caloric and nutrient absorption. This results in a mean of 31.2% TBWL at 1 year and 25.5% TBWL at 5 years.[48] Patients are at risk for vitamin and mineral deficiencies.

Biliopancreatic diversion with duodenal switch (BPD-DS) is a two-step procedure for weight loss. The first is a SG, with the removal of 80% of the stomach, leaving the pyloric valve intact and connected to a small portion of the duodenum. The second step connects the distal small intestine to the duodenal end of the gastric remnant. There is a limited area for ingested food and significantly reduced intestinal surface area for the absorption of nutrients. Patients have a mean of 41% TBWL at 1 year and 37% TBWL at 5 years.[50,51] This surgery has the highest rates of T2DM remission and weight loss but has the greatest risk for malnutrition and vitamin deficiencies of all bariatric surgeries. It is usually performed only in patients with a BMI greater than 50 kg/m^2 or a BMI greater than 40 kg/m^2 with T2DM.

In addition to caloric restriction, SG, RYGB, and BPD-DS usually result in a shift in gastrointestinal hormones in a manner that promotes sustained weight loss, including decreased appetite and increased satiety.[52] In addition to weight loss, hormonal changes may also contribute to the greater improvement and even remission of T2DM compared with intensive lifestyle and medical therapy.[53–56] A recent meta-analysis showed a mean survival benefit of 6 years in bariatric surgery patients compared with those receiving usual care.[57,58]

Postbariatric surgery, patients should be monitored regularly for weight loss, remission of comorbidities, and vitamin/mineral deficiencies.[59] Providers should be aware that weight regain, which has variable definitions, may occur after bariatric surgery. Analysis of data from more than 2000 RYGB surgery patients at multiple medical centers found that 46.9% experienced a weight regain of greater than 15% above nadir postoperative weight at 4 years.[60] A recent single-center study of 445 bariatric surgery patients showed a weight regain of greater than 15% above the nadir postoperative weight occurred in 33.5% of patients at 6 years[61]. Patients with significant weight regain should be evaluated to ensure there are no anatomic/mechanical problems. Refocusing on the appropriate intensive lifestyle interventions appropriate to bariatric surgery should occur as well as monitoring for recurrence of obesity-related comorbidities.

CONTROVERSIES

The noradrenergic agents, like phentermine and diethylpropion, were FDA approved several decades ago, prior to the time when obesity was declared a chronic disease requiring chronic therapy. These medications were approved for 3 months of therapy, unlike the more recently approved antiobesity medications that are approved for chronic therapy. The noradrenergic agents are the only antiobesity medications with generic versions. They are frequently prescribed off-label for longer periods to increase the total amount of weight loss and prevent weight regain, which we expect after discontinuation. Although there are no randomized, double-blind placebo-controlled trials to evaluate the long-term efficacy and safety of these medications,

Table 3
Bariatric surgery

Name	Mean % Total Body Weight Loss at 5 y	Comments	Adverse Events
Laparoscopic adjustable gastric band	12%	• Removable	• Insufficient weight loss • Band slippage • Gastric erosion
Sleeve gastrectomy	19%	• Most commonly performed bariatric surgery	• Gastroesophageal reflux
Roux-en-Y gastric bypass	26%	• Increased technical difficulty compared with sleeve gastrectomy	• Malabsorption of macro-/micronutrients
Biliopancreatic diversion with duodenal switch (BPD-DS)	37%	• Greatest weight loss and metabolic benefits	• Greatest risk for malabsorption of macro-/micronutrients

a large observational study of more than 10,000 patients prescribed phentermine evaluated weight loss and the risk for cardiovascular disease and death with up to 2 years of continuous use. It found that compared with those using phentermine for 3 months, there was a significant increase in weight loss in those using the medication for greater than 3 months, without an increased risk for cardiovascular disease or death with up to 24 months of use.[62]

For all FDA-approved antiobesity medications for chronic therapy, patients should be monitored for response to therapy. As with other medications, some patients may not respond to any particular medication, in which case it should be discontinued or the dose escalated. There are some situations where continuing the medication may be appropriate, even if the weight loss goal has not been met. If a patient experienced progressive weight gain prior to medication initiation and the medication has interrupted this trend, a provider may opt to continue the medication, even if the weight loss goal has not been met. A provider may also consider continuing a medication when the weight loss goal has not been met if it has effectively treated another disorder. For instance, migraine headaches may be treated by phentermine-topiramate or naltrexone-bupropion may have been effective in helping with smoking cessation. Lastly, if a patient has experienced significant weight loss but not reached their weight loss goal on a given medication, the addition of another antiobesity medication may be considered. Although there are no guidelines or large-scale trials supporting such add-on therapy, it is common in clinical practice.

COMPLICATIONS/CONCERNS

The Obesity Society pharmacotherapy guidelines advise that patients be monitored at least monthly during the initial 3 months of pharmacotherapy, and then less frequently if they are stable to assess for medication efficacy and adverse effects. The most common adverse effects of antiobesity medications, devices, and bariatric surgery are detailed in **Tables 1–3**. Patients should be followed closely during the initial year after bariatric surgery to monitor for complications. Further out, patients should be followed at least annually to monitor for complications such as vitamin deficiencies. Bariatric surgery patients may also experience significant weight regain. This may occur due to anatomic complications, such as gastrogastric fistula in patients after RYGB, where a connection develops between the remnant stomach and the smaller gastric pouch, allowing for a greater capacity to ingest food. Decreased adherence to postbariatric surgery dietary, behavior, and activity guidelines may also result in weight regain. Definitions of what constitutes weight regain vary; however, a study by Amundsen, and colleagues found that significant weight regain, defined as greater than 15% above nadir weight, was significantly more likely to occur in those with lower physical activity levels. The group without significant weight regain had a mean of 119 min/d more physical activity than those in the group with significant weight regain.[63] This is why patients should be monitored long term after surgery to reinforce the lifestyle changes that remain the cornerstone for maximizing weight loss and minimizing weight regain postop.

The use of supplements for weight loss is common; however, they are not regulated by the FDA, placing patients at risk of side effects from the declared ingredients or undeclared adulterants.[64–68] The FDA does random testing for a small portion of supplements and often finds that weight loss supplements contain undeclared ingredients. In fact, it is not unusual for testing to find known toxins or medications that have been recalled from the market due to adverse effects.[69]

FUTURE DIRECTIONS

As we learn more about the mechanisms and genetics affecting weight, therapies continue to be developed to target these areas. Several promising therapeutics under development for obesity are described below.

The dual glucose-dependent insulinotropic polypeptide (GIP) and GLP-1R agonist Tirzepatide is currently in phase 3 trials to evaluate efficacy for patients with T2DM compared with placebo.[70] Tirzepatide contains hormonal analogs of the naturally occurring incretin hormones, secreted in response to a meal to increase postprandial insulin production, and also has effects on adipose cells and appetite.[71] A phase 3 open-label trial that evaluated its efficacy in patients with T2DM compared with semaglutide 1 mg found the GIP/GLP-1 receptor agonist was superior to semaglutide 1 mg in reducing hemoglobin A1c levels and reducing body weight.

Bimagrumab is a human monoclonal antibody that binds to a receptor on skeletal muscle, the activin type II receptor. Blockade of the receptor prevents binding of ligands that negatively regulate skeletal muscle growth. A phase 2 trial to evaluate its efficacy in patients with overweight/obesity and T2DM showed that Bimagrumab for 48 weeks decreased total body weight by a mean of 6.5% and decreased total body fat mass by a mean of 20.5%, with 92% of subjects having a $\geq$ 10% decrease in total fat mass. At the same time, lean mass was increased by a mean of 3.6% and hemoglobin A1c decreased by 0.76%.[72]

Setmelanotide is a melanocortin 4 receptor (MC4R) agonist that currently has an orphan drug designation to treat patients with monogenic forms of obesity, including POMC receptor, leptin receptor (LEPR), and pro-protein subtilisin/kexin Type 1 (PCSK1) deficiency, which all result in severe early-onset obesity. Setmelanotide restores activity along the MC4R pathway in the hypothalamus, resulting in decreased appetite and increased energy expenditure. In very small studies of patients with POMC or PCSK1 deficiency treated with setmelanotide, 80% achieved $\geq$ 10% TBWL and 46% of those with LEPR deficiency had $\geq$ 10% TBWL at 1 year.[73] Heterozygous mutations in the MC4R gene are the most common genetic abnormality in those with more common, polygenic, forms of obesity. Heterozygous MC4R mutations have been found in 2%–6% of the general population with early-onset severe obesity.[74–76] Setmelanotide trials continue, and it may be a therapeutic option for patients with common obesity in the future.

Cagrilintide is a long-acting amylin analog currently in trials for obesity therapy. Amylin is a peptide that is co-secreted postprandially with insulin from the pancreas. It suppresses appetite, delays gastric emptying, and suppresses postprandial glucagon release, which result in decreased weight and improved glycemic control. A short-acting form of amylin, pramlintide, is already FDA approved for the therapy of Type 1 and Type 2 diabetes. A 20-week trial with cagrilintide along with semaglutide 2.4 mg (FDA-approved for obesity therapy) resulted in a mean of 17.1% TBWL.[77,78]

Intragastric balloons composed of cellulose hydrogels are currently under development.[79] These do not require an endoscopy for placement or removal, as do current intragastric balloons. Instead, they will break down with a safe calcium solution or after the patient swallows a blue wavelength light capsule.

SUMMARY

Obesity is a disease characterized by metabolic dysfunction, with a variety of contributing factors. These include genetic, epigenetic, social, environmental, and behavioral factors and a complex interplay between adipose tissue, muscle, the gut, and brain, and these connections continue to be elucidated. Our increased understanding of these connections will assist us with the creation of more effective and individualized therapies over time. Although it is currently not possible to determine which therapy will most benefit any individual patient, there are effective medications, devices, and bariatric surgery options, which are able to assist patients in achieving and sustaining weight loss when combined with lifestyle intervention.

CLINICS CARE POINTS

- Obesity is a chronic disease requiring long-term management
- Assess whether chronic medication therapy for other conditions can be adjusted to promote weight loss and achieve sufficient control of the condition
- If BMI is appropriate and patient has been unable to achieve or maintain weight loss, the patient should be considered for additional therapies in a stepwise fashion, including antiobesity medications, medical devices, and bariatric surgery
- Lifestyle changes remain the cornerstone of any other therapies and should be continued as additional therapy is added
- When choosing an antiobesity medication, consider whether it would be useful to also treat another medical condition
- If antiobesity medication is used, monitor for effectiveness and try an alternative if patient does not meet weight loss goals
- If a medication is effective but a patient experiences a weight plateau before reaching their weight loss goal, consider the addition of another medication

DISCLOSURE

T.J. Reid has no relevant financial relationships to disclose. J. Korner is a scientific advisor for Gila Therapeutics.

REFERENCES

1. Hales CM, Carroll MD, Fryar CD, et al. Prevalence of Obesity and Severe Obesity Among Adults: United States, 2017-2018. NCHS Data Brief 2020;(360):1–8.
2. Types of Blood Pressure Medications. 2017. Available at: https://www.heart.org/en/health-topics/high-blood-pressure/changes-you-can-make-to-manage-high-blood-pressure/types-of-blood-pressure-medications. Accessed November 12, 2021.
3. Danek RL, Berlin KL, Waite GN, et al. Perceptions of Nutrition Education in the Current Medical School Curriculum. Fam Med 2017;49(10):803–6.
4. Butsch WS, Kushner RF, Alford S, et al. Low priority of obesity education leads to lack of medical students' preparedness to effectively treat patients with obesity: results from the U.S. medical school obesity education curriculum benchmark study. BMC Med Educ 2020;20(1):23.
5. Butsch WS, Robison K, Sharma R, et al. Medicine Residents are Unprepared to Effectively Treat Patients with Obesity: Results from a U.S. Internal Medicine Residency Survey. J Med Educ Curric Dev 2020;7. 2382120520973206.
6. Dietz WH, Baur LA, Hall K, et al. Management of obesity: improvement of healthcare training and systems for prevention and care. Lancet 2015;385(9986):2521–33.
7. Metcalf M, Rossie K, Stokes K, et al. The perceptions of medical school students and faculty toward obesity medicine education: survey and needs analysis. JMIR Med Educ 2017;3(2):e22.
8. Xia Y, Lelton CML, Guo JJ, et al. Treatment of obesity: pharmacotherapy trends in the United States from 1999 to 2010. Obesity (Silver Spring) 2015;23(8):1721–8.
9. Samaranayake NR, Ong KL, Leung RYH, et al. Management of obesity in the National Health and Nutrition Examination Survey (NHANES), 2007-2008. Ann Epidemiol 2012;22(5):349–53.
10. Kabiri M, Sexton Ward A, Ramasamy A, et al. The societal value of broader access to antiobesity medications. Obesity (Silver Spring) 2020;28(2):429–36.
11. Thomas CE, Elizabeth EA, Shukla AP, et al. Low adoption of weight loss medications: a comparison of prescribing patterns of antiobesity pharmacotherapies and SGLT2s. Obesity (Silver Spring) 2016;24(9):1955–61.
12. Campos GM, Khoraki J, Browning MG, et al. Changes in Utilization of Bariatric Surgery in the United States From 1993 to 2016. Ann Surg 2020;271(2):201–9.
13. Kaplan LM, Golden A, Jinnet K, et al. Perceptions of barriers to effective obesity care: results from the national ACTION Study. Obesity (Silver Spring) 2018;26(1):61–9.
14. English WJ, DeMaria EJ, Hutter MM, et al. American Society for Metabolic and Bariatric Surgery 2018 estimate of metabolic and bariatric procedures performed in the United States. Surg Obes Relat Dis 2020;16(4):457–63.
15. Granara B, Laurent J. Provider attitudes and practice patterns of obesity management with pharmacotherapy. J Am Assoc Nurse Pract 2017;29(9):543–50.
16. Simon R, Lahiri SW. Provider practice habits and barriers to care in obesity management in a large multicenter health system. Endocr Pract 2018;24(4):321–8.
17. Fujioka K, Harris SR. Barriers and Solutions for Prescribing Obesity Pharmacotherapy. Endocrinol Metab Clin North Am 2020;49(2):303–14.
18. Kyle TK, Dhurandhar EJ, Allison DB. Regarding obesity as a disease: evolving policies and their implications. Endocrinol Metab Clin North Am 2016;45(3):511–20.

19. Guh DP, Zhang W, Bansback N, et al. The incidence of co-morbidities related to obesity and overweight: a systematic review and meta-analysis. BMC Public Health 2009;9:88.
20. Oh TJ. The role of anti-obesity medication in prevention of diabetes and its complications. J Obes Metab Syndr 2019;28(3):158–66.
21. Look ARG, Wing RR, Bolin P, et al. Cardiovascular effects of intensive lifestyle intervention in type 2 diabetes. N Engl J Med 2013;369(2):145–54.
22. Goldstein DJ. Beneficial health effects of modest weight loss. Int J Obes Relat Metab Disord 1992;16(6):397–415.
23. Williamson DF. Intentional weight loss: patterns in the general population and its association with morbidity and mortality. Int J Obes Relat Metab Disord 1997; 21(Suppl 1):S14–9 [discussion: S20-S21].
24. Apovian CM, Aronne LJ, Bessesen DH, et al. Pharmacological management of obesity: an endocrine Society clinical practice guideline. J Clin Endocrinol Metab 2015;100(2):342–62.
25. Consultation, W.H.O.E., Appropriate body-mass index for Asian populations and its implications for policy and intervention strategies. Lancet 2004;363(9403): 157–63.
26. Jensen MD, Ryan DH, Apovian CM, et al. 2013 AHA/ACC/TOS guideline for the management of overweight and obesity in adults: a report of the American College of Cardiology/American Heart Association Task Force on Practice Guidelines and The Obesity Society. J Am Coll Cardiol 2014;63(25 Pt B):2985–3023.
27. Khera R, Murad MH, Chandar AK, et al. Association of pharmacological treatments for obesity with weight loss and adverse events: a systematic review and meta-analysis. JAMA 2016;315(22):2424–34.
28. Yanovski SZ, Yanovski JA. Obes N Engl J Med 2002;346(8):591–602.
29. Allison DB, Gadde KM, Garvey WT, et al. Controlled-release phentermine/topiramate in severely obese adults: a randomized controlled trial (EQUIP). Obesity (Silver Spring) 2012;20(2):330–42.
30. Garvey WT, Ryan DH, Look M, et al. Two-year sustained weight loss and metabolic benefits with controlled-release phentermine/topiramate in obese and overweight adults (SEQUEL): a randomized, placebo-controlled, phase 3 extension study. Am J Clin Nutr 2012;95(2):297–308.
31. Davidson MH, Hauptman J, DiGirolamo M, et al. Weight control and risk factor reduction in obese subjects treated for 2 years with orlistat: a randomized controlled trial. JAMA 1999;281(3):235–42.
32. Apovian CM, Aronne L, Rubino D, et al. A randomized, phase 3 trial of naltrexone SR/bupropion SR on weight and obesity-related risk factors (COR-II). Obesity (Silver Spring) 2013;21(5):935–43.
33. Billes SK, Sinnayah P, Cowley MA. Naltrexone/bupropion for obesity: an investigational combination pharmacotherapy for weight loss. Pharmacol Res 2014; 84:1–11.
34. Greenway FL, Fujioka K, Plodkowski RA, et al. Effect of naltrexone plus bupropion on weight loss in overweight and obese adults (COR-I): a multicentre, randomised, double-blind, placebo-controlled, phase 3 trial. Lancet 2010;376(9741): 595–605.
35. Greenway FL, Whitehouse MJ, Guttadauria M, et al. Rational design of a combination medication for the treatment of obesity. Obesity (Silver Spring) 2009; 17(1):30–9.
36. Pi-Sunyer X, Astrup A, Fujioka K, et al. A randomized, controlled trial of 3.0 mg of liraglutide in weight management. N Engl J Med 2015;373(1):11–22.

37. Astrup A, Carraro R, Finer N, et al. Safety, tolerability and sustained weight loss over 2 years with the once-daily human GLP-1 analog, liraglutide. Int J Obes (Lond) 2012;36(6):843–54.
38. Marso SP, Daniels GH, Brown-Frandsen SP, et al. Liraglutide and Cardiovascular Outcomes in Type 2 Diabetes. N Engl J Med 2016;375(4):311–22.
39. Rubino D, Abrahamsson N, Davies M, et al. Effect of continued weekly subcutaneous semaglutide vs placebo on weight loss maintenance in adults with overweight or obesity: The STEP 4 Randomized Clinical Trial. JAMA 2021;325(14): 1414–25.
40. Wadden TA, Bailey TS, Billings LK, et al. Effect of Subcutaneous Semaglutide vs Placebo as an Adjunct to Intensive Behavioral Therapy on Body Weight in Adults With Overweight or Obesity: The STEP 3 Randomized Clinical Trial. JAMA 2021; 325(14):1403–13.
41. Newsome PN, Buchholtz K, Cusi K, et al. A Placebo-Controlled Trial of Subcutaneous Semaglutide in Nonalcoholic Steatohepatitis. N Engl J Med 2021; 384(12):1113–24.
42. Knowler WC, Barrett-Connor E, Fowler SE, et al. Reduction in the incidence of type 2 diabetes with lifestyle intervention or metformin. N Engl J Med 2002; 346(6):393–403.
43. Greenway FL, Aronne LJ, Raben A, et al. A randomized, double-blind, placebo-controlled study of Gelesis100: a novel nonsystemic oral hydrogel for weight loss. Obesity (Silver Spring) 2019;27(2):205–16.
44. Imaz I, Martinez-Cervell C, Garcia-Alvarez EE, et al. Safety and effectiveness of the intragastric balloon for obesity. A meta-analysis. Obes Surg 2008;18(7): 841–6.
45. Gaur S, Levy S, Mathus-Vliegen L, et al. Balancing risk and reward: a critical review of the intragastric balloon for weight loss. Gastrointest Endosc 2015;81(6): 1330–6.
46. Herve J, Wahlen CH, Schaeken A, et al. What becomes of patients one year after the intragastric balloon has been removed? Obes Surg 2005;15(6):864–70.
47. Thompson CC, Abu Dayyeh BK, Kushner R, et al. Percutaneous gastrostomy device for the treatment of Class II and Class III Obesity: results of a randomized controlled trial. Am J Gastroenterol 2017;112(3):447–57.
48. Arterburn D, Wellman R, Emiliano A, et al. Comparative effectiveness and safety of bariatric procedures for weight loss: A PCORnet Cohort Study. Ann Intern Med 2018;169(11):741–50.
49. Park CH, Nam S, Choi HS, et al. Comparative efficacy of bariatric surgery in the treatment of morbid obesity and diabetes mellitus: a systematic review and network meta-analysis. Obes Surg 2019;29(7):2180–90.
50. Marinari GM, Papadia FS, Briatore L, et al. Type 2 diabetes and weight loss following biliopancreatic diversion for obesity. Obes Surg 2006;16(11):1440–4.
51. Topart P, Becouarn G, Delarue J. Weight loss and nutritional outcomes 10 years after biliopancreatic diversion with duodenal switch. Obes Surg 2017;27(7): 1645–50.
52. Papamargaritis D, le Roux CW. Do Gut Hormones Contribute to Weight Loss and Glycaemic Outcomes after Bariatric Surgery? Nutrients 2021;13(3).
53. Ikramuddin S, Korner J, Lee WJ, et al. Lifestyle Intervention and Medical Management With vs Without Roux-en-Y Gastric Bypass and Control of Hemoglobin A1c, LDL Cholesterol, and Systolic Blood Pressure at 5 Years in the Diabetes Surgery Study. JAMA 2018;319(3):266–78.

54. Mingrone G, Panunzi S, De Gaetano A, et al. Metabolic surgery versus conventional medical therapy in patients with type 2 diabetes: 10-year follow-up of an open-label, single-centre, randomised controlled trial. Lancet 2021;397(10271): 293–304.

55. Arterburn DE, Telem DA, Kushner RF, et al. Benefits and risks of bariatric surgery in adults: a review. JAMA 2020;324(9):879–87.

56. Nguyen KT, Korner J. The sum of many parts: potential mechanisms for improvement in glucose homeostasis after bariatric surgery. Curr Diab Rep 2014; 14(5):481.

57. Syn NL, Cummings DE, Wang LZ, et al. Association of metabolic-bariatric surgery with long-term survival in adults with and without diabetes: a one-stage meta-analysis of matched cohort and prospective controlled studies with 174 772 participants. Lancet 2021;397(10287):1830–41.

58. Aminian A, Scarfo P, Lochy S, et al. Association of bariatric surgery with major adverse liver and cardiovascular outcomes in patients with biopsy-proven nonalcoholic steatohepatitis. JAMA 2021;326(20):2031–42.

59. Parrott J, Frank L, Rabena R, et al. American Society for Metabolic and Bariatric Surgery Integrated Health Nutritional Guidelines for the Surgical Weight Loss Patient 2016 Update: Micronutrients. Surg Obes Relat Dis 2017;13(5):727–41.

60. King WC, Hinerman AS, Belle SH, et al. Comparison of the Performance of Common Measures of Weight Regain After Bariatric Surgery for Association With Clinical Outcomes. JAMA 2018;320(15):1560–9.

61. Torrego-Ellacuria M, Torrego-Ellacuría M, Del Rey-Mejías, et al. Weight regain outcomes after bariatric surgery in the long-term follow-up: role of preoperative factors. Obes Surg 2021;31(9):3947–55.

62. Lewis KH, Fischer H, Ard J, et al. Safety and effectiveness of longer-term phentermine use: clinical outcomes from an electronic health record cohort. Obesity (Silver Spring) 2019;27(4):591–602.

63. Amundsen T, Strommen M, Martins C. Suboptimal weight loss and weight regain after gastric bypass surgery-postoperative status of energy intake, eating behavior, physical activity, and psychometrics. Obes Surg 2017;27(5):1316–23.

64. Chitturi S, Farrell GC. Hepatotoxic slimming aids and other herbal hepatotoxins. J Gastroenterol Hepatol 2008;23(3):366–73.

65. De Smet PA. Herbal remedies. N Engl J Med 2002;347(25):2046–56.

66. Cohen PA. American roulette–contaminated dietary supplements. N Engl J Med 2009;361(16):1523–5.

67. Parker ML, Stefan C, Reich HN, et al. What Is Really in This Weight Loss Supplement? J Appl Lab Med 2019;4(2):270–3.

68. Pittler MH, Schmidt K, Ernst E. Adverse events of herbal food supplements for body weight reduction: systematic review. Obes Rev 2005;6(2):93–111.

69. FDA Recalls, Market Withdrawals, & Safety Alerts. 2021. Available at: https://www.fda.gov/safety/recalls-market-withdrawals-safety-alerts. Accessed December 21, 2021.

70. Frias JP, Davies MJ, Rosenstock J, et al. Tirzepatide versus Semaglutide Once Weekly in Patients with Type 2 Diabetes. N Engl J Med 2021;385(6):503–15.

71. Nauck MA, Meier JJ. Incretin hormones: Their role in health and disease. Diabetes Obes Metab 2018;20(Suppl 1):5–21.

72. Heymsfield SB, Coleman LA, Miller R, et al. Effect of Bimagrumab vs Placebo on Body Fat Mass Among Adults With Type 2 Diabetes and Obesity: A Phase 2 Randomized Clinical Trial. JAMA Netw Open 2021;4(1):e2033457.

73. Clement K, van den Akker E, Argente J, et al. Efficacy and safety of setmelano-tide, an MC4R agonist, in individuals with severe obesity due to LEPR or POMC deficiency: single-arm, open-label, multicentre, phase 3 trials. Lancet Diabetes Endocrinol 2020;8(12):960–70.
74. Calton MA, Ersoy BA, Zhang S, et al. Association of functionally significant Melanocortin-4 but not Melanocortin-3 receptor mutations with severe adult obesity in a large North American case-control study. Hum Mol Genet 2009; 18(6):1140–7.
75. Farooqi IS, Keogh JM, Yeo GS, et al. Clinical spectrum of obesity and mutations in the melanocortin 4 receptor gene. N Engl J Med 2003;348(12):1085–95.
76. Hinney A, Hohmann S, Geller F, et al. Melanocortin-4 receptor gene: case-control study and transmission disequilibrium test confirm that functionally relevant mutations are compatible with a major gene effect for extreme obesity. J Clin Endocrinol Metab 2003;88(9):4258–67.
77. Becerril S, Fruhbeck G. Cagrilintide plus semaglutide for obesity management. Lancet 2021;397(10286):1687–9.
78. Enebo LB, Berthelsen KK, Kankam M, et al. Safety, tolerability, pharmacokinetics, and pharmacodynamics of concomitant administration of multiple doses of cagrilintide with semaglutide 2.4 mg for weight management: a randomised, controlled, phase 1b trial. Lancet 2021;397(10286):1736–48.
79. Liu X, Steiger C, Lin S, et al. Ingestible hydrogel device. Nat Commun 2019; 10(1):493.

Nutritional Aspects of Healthy Aging

Alexander Panda, MD, PhD, MPH, Sarah L. Booth, PhD*

KEYWORDS

- Aging • Nutrition • Dietary requirements • Healthspan

KEY POINTS

- Older adults are susceptible to nutritional or dietary deficiencies that can lead to or exacerbate age-related declines in physical, physiologic, and cognitive function.
- In older age, loss of appetite and decreased food intake accompany a decrease in energy needs. However, the decreased energy requirements are not always offset by reduced appetite.
- Micronutrient requirements remain the same or increase in older age, so it is particularly important for older adults to consume nutrient-dense foods.
- Older adults are prone to under-hydration yet they may not feel thirsty, so adequate water intake should also be encouraged.

INTRODUCTION

Over the next 3 decades, the number of older persons is projected to more than double globally, reaching more than 1.5 billion persons by 2050.[1] More than 46 million older adults aged 65 years and older are living in the US today, and this number is expected to grow to almost 90 million by 2050.[2]

Aging is characterized by a continuum of various physical, physiologic, and cognitive changes. Multiple theories explain the mechanisms of aging at the system, biologic, cellular, and molecular levels.[3] Of these, the programmed theories propose a biological timetable driven by changes in gene expression which affects maintenance, repair, and defense mechanisms. In contrast, the damage and error theory focus on environmental impacts that result in cumulative changes on biologic, cellular, and molecular levels. Cumulatively, these factors influence both lifespan and healthspan. There is a recognized gap between lifespan, which is defined as the total life lived, and healthspan, which is defined as the period free from disease.[4] Using health-adjusted life expectancy that takes into consideration life expectancy, years lived

Jean Mayer USDA Human Nutrition Research Center on Aging, Tufts University, 711 Washington Street, Boston, MA 02111, USA
* Corresponding author.
E-mail address: sarah.booth@tufts.edu

Med Clin N Am 106 (2022) 853–863
https://doi.org/10.1016/j.mcna.2022.04.008
0025-7125/22/© 2022 Elsevier Inc. All rights reserved.

medical.theclinics.com

with disability, and premature death from disease, the healthspan to lifespan gap is estimated at around 9 years.[5,6] This has important implications for the current health care system given the increasing numbers of older individuals experiencing longer years with disabilities and requiring medical care.

Nutrition and healthy eating habits are key determinants for extending healthspan. They are readily modifiable interventions and can promote optimal health and well-being in older adults. Like aging, the nutritional decline in the elderly is multifactorial ranging from physiologic and metabolic changes to socioeconomic barriers and disparities and isolation as people transition into a less active lifestyle after retirement.[7–9] In this article, we will focus on the physiologic and metabolic issues, and present practical guidance based on current knowledge regarding dietary guidance for older adults.

DISCUSSION
Physiologic Decline in Food intake with Aging

Aging is characterized by loss of appetite resulting in decreased food intake. There can also be a decreased ability to ingest adequate amount of food. An excess decline in food intake can lead to weight loss, and contribute to muscle wasting and frailty, decreased function of respiratory muscles, impaired immune function with depressed antibody and cell-mediated responses and consequent greater susceptibility to infections, reduced gut function, and increased bacterial translocation.[10] The correlation between age-related nutritional deficits with multiple adverse outcomes has been well described and is referred to as "anorexia of aging."[11] It is often overseen by the treating physician or mistakenly assumed to be a normal aspect of aging, whereas anorexia of aging is a true geriatric syndrome that affects up to 30% of older persons.

A multitude of factors contributes to decreased food intake and anorexia of aging.[12,13] Several hormones such as cholecystokinin (CCK), ghrelin, leptin, insulin, glucagon-like peptide-1 and peptide YY (PYY) play an important role in nutritional changes in aging. Evidence suggests that with advancing age, there is an increase in satiety hormones, such as CCK and PYY, and a decrease in the hunger hormone, ghrelin, which regulates food intake by enhancing gastric emptying.[14] Low ghrelin plasma levels result in delayed gastric emptying, and when combined with increased satiety, contributes to decreased food intake. In addition, increased circulating leptin levels and low insulin levels are also associated with anorexia in older adults. Inflamm-aging, the chronic low-grade inflammation that develops with advanced age, is not only responsible for the increased susceptibility of the elderly to infectious diseases but higher levels of proinflammatory cytokines such as Interleukin (IL) 1, IL6 and Tumor Necrosis Factor-alpha (TNK-α) have also been linked to delayed gastric emptying and the increase of leptin levels, which in turn reduce food intake.[15,16]

Smell and taste also decline with aging, and even further deteriorate when nutritional deficiencies occur.[17] Furthermore, oral health is an important factor directly impacting the quality and amount of food intake. Almost 19% of older adults no longer have natural teeth. Adults aged 75 years and older are twice as likely to be edentulous as those aged 65 to 74 years (13%). Non-Hispanic Blacks (29%) were significantly more likely to be edentulous compared with Hispanics (15%) and non-Hispanic Whites (17%).[18] A Massachusetts survey revealed that 34% of seniors in nursing homes have urgent and major dental health needs.[19] A logical consequence of poor dentition is the consumption of less nutritious, soft, easily chewable food as compared with fresh fruits or vegetables. Xerostomia (dry mouth) due to hyposalivation often aggregates this condition and increases the likelihood of infections within the oral cavity worsening the nutritional decline even more and contributing to the poor nutritional status of many elderly.[14,20]

Nutrient Needs for Older Adults

General concepts

In the US, nutritional requirements, called Dietary Reference Intakes (DRI), have been established for healthy, normal-weight individuals across the lifespan.[21] Limited scientific evidence is currently available on the nutritional requirements for older adults, especially those considered the oldest old (ie, currently defined as those more than 80 years of age). This does present challenges when designing optimal diets for older adults because the original framework for developing individual DRIs assumes normal weight and free of disease. In contrast, approximately one-third of US elderly are currently considered obese and 85% of all older adults have at least one chronic disease. How these diseases impact the nutritional needs of older adults are not well understood, in part because most research on nutritional requirements exclude individuals with chronic diseases. The National Academies of Sciences, Engineering, and Medicine (NASEM; formerly known as the Institute of Medicine) recently revised their approach to include the concept of chronic disease reduction when updating DRIs.[22] Thus far, this revised framework has only been applied to sodium and potassium.[23] For most nutrients, the requirements are extrapolated from data generated in healthy, normal-weight adults, ages 19 to 50 years of age.

Dietary energy

Concurrent with the decrease in appetite and food intake associated with aging, there is also a large decrease in dietary energy needs as individuals' age. Recent data examining energy expenditure over the life course suggest that overall dietary energy required to maintain healthy weight is stable between the ages of 20 and 60 years of age, after which there are marked decreases in healthy women and men.[24] Very little data exist for those in the oldest old age category so it is unclear if this negative trajectory of energy changes its slope at the end of the lifespan. These decreased energy requirements are not always offset by reduced appetite. Indeed, obesity is a significant problem among the elderly, which itself is a risk factor for frailty for both men and women.[25] In the context of decreasing energy needs, the absolute intake of protein and certain micronutrients needs to be stable or increased in certain circumstances, as discussed later in discussion, thereby emphasizing the need for nutrient-dense foods for older adults.

Dietary energy needs also vary depending on sex and activity level. Inactive adults—defined as getting less than 30 minutes per day of physical activity—need fewer calories than adults who are moderately active (between 30 and 45 minutes of activity per day) or active (more than 45 minutes per day), according to the United States Department of Agriculture (USDA).[26] At the time of this writing, National Academies of Sciences, Engineering, and Medicine (NASEM) was convening an ad hoc committee to reassess the human requirements for energy intake and expenditure, including energy requirements to support recovery from disease and treatments or interventions such as surgery.

Macronutrients

The currently recommended proportions of dietary energy from intake of fat and carbohydrates are unchanged with aging. The current guidance for dietary fat is a balanced diet of 20% to 35% energy as fat, particularly high in monosaturated and polyunsaturated fats (linoleic acid [n-6] [g/d]: 5% to 10% and alpha-linolenic Acid [n-3] [g/d]: 0.6%–1.2%), reduced intake of dietary cholesterol and saturated fat, and no trans-fatty acids.[21,27] About 60% percent of dietary energy come from carbohydrates, with emphasis on complex carbohydrates. Glucose tolerance may decrease with advancing years, and complex carbohydrates put less stress on maintaining circulating blood glucose compared with refined carbohydrates.[28]

Many older adults do not meet recommended intake of protein. This, in combination with other factors such as inflammation may result in loss of muscle loss, a condition known as sarcopenia. About 30% of individuals aged 60 years and above are sarcopenic, while more than 50% of individuals aged 80 years and older are estimated to be sarcopenic.[29] Current guidance is that older adults need to consume at least the same protein intakes as those younger adults, and a common formula to calculate daily protein intake is weight in kg multiplied by 0.8. According to this formula, a 70 kg healthy male should consume 56 mg of protein.[21] However, this is somewhat controversial, and some studies indicate that a protein intake of 1.3 to 1.73 g/kg/day is necessary for better health status as compared with to the currently recommended intake of 0.8 g/kg/d [29] Others conclude that protein intake of 1.2 g/kg/d provides adequate calcium homeostasis required for bone health.[30] The optimal amount of protein required during acute illness is not known. Completion of randomized trials, such as the planned NUTRIREA-3 trial, which is a randomized, controlled, multicenter, open-label trial designed to compare standard calorie and protein feeding with a low calorie, low protein feeding in acute illness,[31] are necessary for addressing this important gap in knowledge. .

Dehydration is the most common fluid or electrolyte disturbance in older adults, yet water intake has often been overlooked in nutrition and health research. Recent evidence links under-hydration and habitual low water intake to higher cardiometabolic risk in community-dwelling older adults.[32] There seems to be a consistent pattern between circulating lipid concentrations and different water sources and hydration markers supporting an association between hydration and lipid metabolism in older adults, thus adding to the growing evidence to support the theory that inadequate water intake and under-hydration may lead to higher cardiometabolic risk. Generally, older adults require 30 mL/kg/d or 1 mL/kcal ingested (2–4 L) fluids per day. Fluid needs to increase with fever, infection, or with diuretic or laxative therapy. Recommended fluids include water and unsweetened beverages with no or low caloric value to avoid consumption of excess calories. Adequate water intake also reduces stress on kidney function, which tends to decline with age, and eases constipation. With the aging process, the ability to detect thirst declines, so frequent water intake is encouraged. Caution regarding water intake though must be exercised in elderly with thyroid disease or specific kidney, liver, or heart problems, or when taking medications that potentially can lead to the retention of water, such as nonsteroidal anti-inflammatory drugs (NSAIDs), opiate pain medications, and some antidepressants.[33]

Adequate dietary fiber, together with adequate fluid, helps maintain normal bowel function. Fiber also is thought to decrease the risk of intestinal inflammation. Current daily fiber recommendations for those aged 50 years or older are at least 30 g for men and 21 g for women, or at minimum 14 g of fiber per 1000 kcal.[21] These recommended total dietary fiber intakes are lower than younger age groups due to the lower recommended calorie intakes. There are multiple types of dietary fiber, and the putative beneficial mechanisms relate to the degree of fermentability and viscosity in the gastrointestinal tract.[34] High fiber diets decreases appetite by decreasing the gastric emptying time, although recent data using SmartPill technology suggest that both food form and fiber content should be taken into account because gastric emptying is much longer in response to a solid test meal compared with a liquid test meal.[35] High fiber diets also improve glycemic control and reduce cholesterol; increased fiber intake has been associated with decreased all-cause mortality, decreased incidence of diabetes, type 2, coronary artery disease, and colorectal cancer.[36] Fiber-rich foods often have higher nutrient composition and lead to increased satiety. Of note, particularly to the clinician, when recommending the increase of fiber content in the diet of an older adult, fluid requirements must also be assessed.

Micronutrients

With fewer total daily calories required to maintain a healthy weight among older adults, it is a challenge to achieve the same micronutrient requirements as younger adults while consuming less food. This is complicated by decreased bioavailability, absorption, and storage of vitamins and minerals with aging, coupled with declining renal function and often undiagnosed gastrointestinal conditions, such as atrophic gastritis. These targets can be overall met by: (1) consuming more nutrient-dense foods, which are foods rich in nutrients relative to their caloric content; and (2) removing proportionally more foods and beverages that contain calories but no or few nutrients than is required for younger adults to maintain a healthy weight. However, this is a considered challenge for which little guidance is available. Indeed, a recent report by the Government Accounting Office concluded that federal agencies need to do more to meet the nutritional needs of older adults, particularly those participating in nutritional assistance programs.[37] As previously stated, micronutrient requirements have also been relatively understudied among older adults, in part to the challenges of designing robust studies among older adults who are heterogenous in their rate of aging and disease states. In that context, here we focus on those micronutrients for which there is evidence of specific concerns in meeting dietary requirements among older adults, specifically vitamins D and calcium, B6, B12, and iron. We also summarize the new chronic disease-specific sodium and potassium recommendations.

Vitamin D and calcium. The current recommendations are 800 IU per day of vitamin D for adults more than 70 years of age, which is higher than younger age groups and is based on strong scientific evidence to support bone health.[38] Similarly, calcium intake recommendations for women aged 51 and older are 1200 mg of calcium per day, which are higher than younger age groups. Calcium recommendations for men aged 50 to 70 years of age are 1000 mg a day and 1200 mg a day for those more than 70 years.[38]

More than 1.5 million fractures are reported each year in individuals more than the age of 60 in the United States alone. Several recent meta-analyses have confirmed the benefits of calcium and vitamin D to reduce hip fracture risk. The active vitamin D metabolite 1,25(OH)2D stimulates the absorption of calcium from the gut. The consequences of vitamin D deficiency are secondary hyperparathyroidism and bone loss, leading to osteoporosis and fractures, mineralization defects, which may potentially lead to osteomalacia, and muscle weakness, causing falls and fractures.[39] There are some more recent data to suggest that this level of intake may also reduce risk of acute respiratory infection in older adults.[40] Older people frequently present with vitamin D deficiency, which is still considered a global challenge, and calcium recommended intakes are only met in Northern European countries.[41] While there has been some speculation that vitamin D and calcium supplements can contribute to cardiovascular disease or all-cause mortality, the preponderance of evidence does not support this claim.[30]

Vitamin B6 (pyridoxine). For adults more than the age of 50, the recommended daily amount of vitamin B6 is 1.5 mg for women and 1.7 mg for men.[42] Vitamin B6 in coenzyme forms performs a wide variety of functions in the body. It is extremely versatile, with involvement in more than 100 enzyme reactions, and is important for cognitive development through the biosynthesis of neurotransmitters and in maintaining normal levels of homocysteine. People who have kidney disease or conditions that prevent the small intestine from absorbing nutrients from foods (malabsorption syndromes) are more likely to be vitamin B-6 deficient. Certain autoimmune disorders, some epilepsy medications, and alcohol dependence also can lead to vitamin B-6 deficiency, leading to macrocytic anemia, depression, and weakened immune system. Of note, vitamin B-6 deficiency is usually coupled with deficiency in other B vitamins, such as folic acid (vitamin B-9) and vitamin B-12.

Vitamin B12 (cobalamin). Vitamin B12 is required for the development, myelination, and function of the central nervous system; healthy red blood cell formation; and DNA synthesis. Current daily recommendations for B12 are 2.4 mcg for all adults, regardless of age.[42] 3% and 43% of community-dwelling older adults have vitamin B12 deficiency based on serum vitamin B12 levels. The deficiency often goes unnoticed because the clinical manifestations are highly variable, often subtle, and nonspecific, but if left undiagnosed the consequences can be serious.[43,44] Conditions associated with vitamin B12 inadequacy include pernicious anemia, present in about 15% to 25% of older adults with vitamin B12 deficiency. Atrophic gastritis, an autoimmune condition affecting 2% of the general population but 8% to 9% of adults aged 65 and older, decreases the production of intrinsic factor and secretion of hydrochloric acid in the stomach and thus decreases the absorption of vitamin B12.[45,46] Another condition associated with vitamin B12 deficiency in older adults is Helicobacter pylori infection, likely because this bacterium causes inflammation that leads to the malabsorption of vitamin B12 from food. Vitamin B12 is a water-soluble vitamin that is naturally present in some foods, added to others, and available as a dietary supplement and a prescription medication.

Iron. Dietary iron has 2 main forms: heme and nonheme. Plants and iron-fortified foods contain nonheme iron only, whereas meat, seafood, and poultry contain both heme and nonheme iron.[47] Iron deficiency is common in the elderly and progresses from the depletion of iron stores (mild iron deficiency) to iron-deficiency erythropoiesis (erythrocyte production), and finally to iron deficiency anemia. About 10% of adults more than 65 are anemic, a number that increases to 20% for those more than 85. Both of these numbers are even higher for those in assisted living homes.[48] Anemia in the elderly is a common finding that is associated with a poorer quality of life, worse outcomes, and increased mortality. Because iron deficiency is often accompanied by deficiencies of other nutrients, the signs and symptoms of iron deficiency can be difficult to isolate. The current recommended daily intake of iron is 8 mg for women and men more than the age of 50 years.[49]

Sodium and potassium. In 2019, NASEM revised the DRIs for sodium and potassium to include the concept of chronic disease reduction when updating DRIs.[23] The adequate intake for sodium for people 14 years and older is 1500 mg/d, whereas the chronic disease risk reduction intake level recommendation is to limit intake to <2300 mg/d. Of note, the 2300 mg/d level is intended to be interpreted as an upper tolerable level, not a target. For potassium, the current daily recommendations are 3400 mg and 2600 mg for men and women, respectively. The most recent estimates from NHANES suggest that only 26.2% of US adults consume sodium less than 2300 mg/d and only 36.0% of men and 38.1% of women meet the dietary requirements for potassium.[50] This pattern of consuming too much sodium and too little potassium is of concern because sodium to potassium of >1.0 is associated with increased risk for cardiovascular disease, particularly among those with hypertension.[51] Similarly, there is some suggestion that too low a sodium intake can also be associated with a higher risk of cardiovascular events and mortality.

Dietary Recommendations Promoting Healthy Aging

There is a preponderance of different dietary patterns that have claims of superiority in promoting healthy aging. The majority have not been rigorously studied to confirm their claims of efficacy, and it is beyond the scope of this review to evaluate each of the more popular dietary patterns and diet plans. In contrast, the Dietary Guidelines for Americans (DGAs) are issued at least every 5 years, and provide food and beverage guidance based on the most current scientific data to support health.[52] In preparation for the most recent DGAs issued in 2020, a systematic review of 1 randomized clinical trial and 152 observational studies concluded that dietary patterns with high intake of fruits and vegetables, legumes, nuts, and whole grains, unsaturated vegetable oils, fish and lean meat and low intake of red and processed meat, high-fat dairy, and refined carbohydrates among older adults were associated with lower mortality risk.[53] The research team concluded that such dietary patterns were rich in nutrient-dense foods, which is critical for older adults who have similar if not higher micronutrient requirements than younger adults but lower dietary energy needs. A similar conclusion was made in the 2021 American Heart Association's Dietary Guidance to Improve Cardiovascular Health.[54] There is a controversy that current recommendations, including the DGAs, are over-simplistic in that one set of recommendations cannot address the large inter-individual variability in response to specific foods and beverages. However, the field of personalized or precision nutrition is still in its infancy and until the factors determining the individual response to different dietary patterns are better elucidated, the DGAs are still the best practical guidance for older adults seeking healthy dietary patterns.[52]

As reviewed elsewhere,[55] older adults, in general, consume below-recommended portions of most healthy nutrient-dense food groups, whereas they consume excess amounts of meats, saturated fats, and added sugars compared with the recommendations. To assist older adults in making better food and beverage choices, researchers at Tufts University developed the MyPlate for Older Adults as a tool to provide practical food and beverage guidance that is specifically tailored for older adults.[56] The most recent version reflects the 2015 to 2020 DGA guidance[57] (Fig. 1). Depicted as a dinner plate, the guidance recommends that half the plate should contain fruits and vegetables in forms that are convenient, affordable, and accessible, such as frozen, prepeeled fresh, dried, and certain low-sodium, low-sugar canned options. Both within the vegetable group and the fruit group, selection of foods that span a variety of deep colors, such as green, orange, red or yellow, are recommended to best meet multiple micronutrient and dietary fiber needs. Liquid vegetable oils are recommended in small amounts consistent with recent guidance for a heart-healthy diet[54] and the recommendation to use herbs and spices in lieu of salt is given that most of the older adults need to reduce their sodium intake. Adequate fluid intake is encouraged with an emphasis on those beverages that are not high in calories, such as water and unsweetened tea. Low-fat dairy products represent a small portion of the plate and provide protein, calcium, and other nutrients while avoiding the higher calorie content of full-fat dairy products. Protein and grain recommendations are consistent with the current 2020 DGAs,[52] with an emphasis on lean meats, nuts and fish, and whole grains. These general principles can be adapted to accommodate different cultural and food preferences.

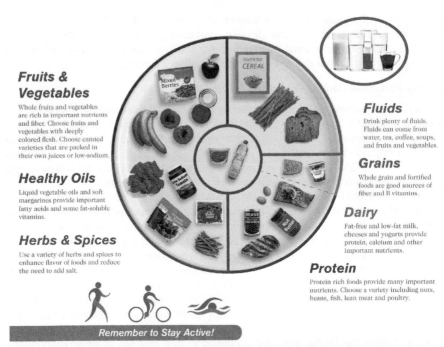

Fruits & Vegetables

Whole fruits and vegetables are rich in important nutrients and fiber. Choose fruits and vegetables with deeply colored flesh. Choose canned varieties that are packed in their own juices or low-sodium.

Healthy Oils

Liquid vegetable oils and soft margarines provide important fatty acids and some fat-soluble vitamins.

Herbs & Spices

Use a variety of herbs and spices to enhance flavor of foods and reduce the need to add salt.

Fluids

Drink plenty of fluids. Fluids can come from water, tea, coffee, soups, and fruits and vegetables.

Grains

Whole grain and fortified foods are good sources of fiber and B vitamins.

Dairy

Fat-free and low-fat milk, cheeses and yogurts provide protein, calcium and other important nutrients.

Protein

Protein rich foods provide many important nutrients. Choose a variety including nuts, beans, fish, lean meat and poultry.

Remember to Stay Active!

Fig. 1. My plate for older adults. "My Plate for Older Adults" Copyright 2016 Tufts University, all rights reserved. "My Plate for Older Adults" graphic and accompanying website were developed with support from the AARP Foundation. "Tufts University" and "AARP Foundation" are registered trademarks and may not be reproduced apart from their inclusion in the "My Plate for Older Adults" graphic without express permission from their respective owners.

SUMMARY

Healthy eating habits may help promote optimal health and well-being in older adults. While there are many gaps in our understanding of how nutritional requirements change with aging, particularly among the oldest old, current guidance to consume nutrient-dense foods while limiting those foods and beverages that contribute calories across the lifespan also applies to older adults. Indeed, as dietary energy needs decline in the older adult, on average their micronutrient needs either remain the same or increase, the concept of nutrient density is believed critical for emphasis when providing dietary guidance for this age group. Fluid intake is also an important concept because this age group is vulnerable to underhydration. Unfortunately, the majority of older adults do not meet the recommended dietary guidance and many have multiple chronic diseases, for which there is inadequate understanding of how the individual chronic diseases and their associated treatments impact dietary guidance.

CLINICS CARE POINTS

- Anorexia of aging is a geriatric syndrome that affects up to 30% of older persons, and should not be assumed to be normal aging, which is characterized by loss of appetite resulting in decreased food intake commensurate with lower dietary energy needs.

- Older adults need to consume more nutrient-dense foods compared with younger adults to maintain a healthy weight and meet their micronutrient needs.
- Fluid intake is often inadequate and when increased fluid intake is required, water should be the beverage of choice as it does not contain calories.

DISCLOSURE

Neither author has any commercial or financial conflicts of interest. This work was supported by the USDA Agricultural Research Service under Cooperative Agreement No. 58-8050-9-004. Any opinions, findings, conclusions, or recommendations expressed in this publication are those of the authors and do not necessarily reflect the views of the USDA.

REFERENCES

1. United Nations. World population ageing 2019 highlights. In: Department of economic and social affairs PD. United Nations; 2019.
2. Bureau USC. Older population and aging. 2021. Available at: https://www.census.gov/topics/population/older-aging.html. Accessed December 10, 2021.
3. Katcher HL. Towards an evidence-based model of aging. Curr Aging Sci 2015; 8(1):46–55.
4. Garmany A, Yamada S, Terzic A. Longevity leap: mind the healthspan gap. NPJ Regen Med 2021;6(1):57.
5. Olshansky SJ. From Lifespan to healthspan. JAMA 2018;320(13):1323–4.
6. Geneva: World Health Organization; 2020.
7. Kaur D, Rasane P, Singh J, et al. Nutritional interventions for elderly and considerations for the development of geriatric foods. Curr Aging Sci 2019;12(1):15–27.
8. Anton SD, Hida A, Mankowski R, et al. Nutrition and exercise in sarcopenia. Curr Protein Pept Sci 2018;19(7):649–67.
9. Hsieh TJ, Chang HY, Wu IC, et al. Independent association between subjective cognitive decline and frailty in the elderly. PLoS One 2018;13(8):e0201351.
10. Chapman IM, MacIntosh CG, Morley JE, et al. The anorexia of ageing. Biogerontology 2002;3(1–2):67–71.
11. Landi F, Picca A, Calvani R, et al. Anorexia of aging: assessment and management. Clin Geriatr Med 2017;33(3):315–23.
12. Visvanathan R. Anorexia of aging. Clin Geriatr Med 2015;31(3):417–27.
13. de Boer A, Ter Horst GJ, Lorist MM. Physiological and psychosocial age-related changes associated with reduced food intake in older persons. Ageing Res Rev 2013;12(1):316–28.
14. Landi F, Calvani R, Tosato M, et al. Anorexia of aging: risk factors, consequences, and potential treatments. Nutrients 2016;8(2):69.
15. Martone AM, Onder G, Vetrano DL, et al. Anorexia of aging: a modifiable risk factor for frailty. Nutrients 2013;5(10):4126–33.
16. Shaw AC, Goldstein DR, Montgomery RR. Age-dependent dysregulation of innate immunity. Nat Rev Immunol 2013;13(12):875–87.
17. Bigman G. Age-related smell and taste impairments and vitamin d associations in the u.s. adults national health and nutrition examination survey. Nutrients 2020;12(4).
18. Dye B, Thorton-Evans G, Li X, et al. Dental caries and tooth loss in adults in the United States, 2011–2012. NCHS Data Brief 2015;197.

19. Trusts PC. A path to expanded dental access in Massachusetts. Philadelphia, PA 2015.
20. Turner MD, Ship JA. Dry mouth and its effects on the oral health of elderly people. J Am Dent Assoc 2007;138(Suppl):15S–20S.
21. Institute of Medicine Food and Nutrition Board. Dietary reference intakes for energy, carbohydrate, fiber, fatty acids, cholesterol, protein and amino acids. Washington, DC 2002.
22. In: Oria MP, Kumanyika S, eds. Guiding principles for developing dietary reference intakes based on chronic disease. Washington, DC 2017.
23. In: Oria M, Harrison M, Stallings VA, eds. Dietary reference intakes for sodium and potassium. Washington, DC 2019.
24. Pontzer H, Yamada Y, Sagayama H, et al. Daily energy expenditure through the human life course. Science 2021;373(6556):808–12.
25. Jensen GL, Friedmann JM. Obesity is associated with functional decline in community-dwelling rural older persons. J Am Geriatr Soc 2002;50(5):918–23.
26. https://www.fns.usda.gov/estimated-calorie-needs-day-age-gender-and-physical-activity-level (Accessed10 December 2021).
27. Gonzalez-Campoy JM, St Jeor ST, Castorino K, et al. Clinical practice guidelines for healthy eating for the prevention and treatment of metabolic and endocrine diseases in adults: cosponsored by the American association of clinical endocrinologists/the american college of endocrinology and the obesity society. Endocr Pract 2013;19(Suppl 3):1–82.
28. Hall KD, Ayuketah A, Brychta R, et al. Ultra-processed diets cause excess calorie intake and weight gain: an inpatient randomized controlled trial of ad libitum food intake. Cell Metab 2019;30(1):226.
29. Gaffney-Stomberg E, Insogna KL, Rodriguez NR, et al. Increasing dietary protein requirements in elderly people for optimal muscle and bone health. J Am Geriatr Soc 2009;57(6):1073–9.
30. Anam AK, Insogna K. Update on osteoporosis screening and management. Med Clin North Am 2021;105(6):1117–34.
31. Reignier J, Le Gouge A, Lascarrou JB, et al. Impact of early low-calorie low-protein versus standard-calorie standard-protein feeding on outcomes of ventilated adults with shock: design and conduct of a randomised, controlled, multicentre, open-label, parallel-group trial (NUTRIREA-3). BMJ Open 2021;11(5):e045041.
32. Jacques PF, Rogers G, Stookey JD, et al. Water intake and markers of hydration are related to cardiometabolic risk biomarkers in community-dwelling older adults: a cross-sectional analysis. J Nutr 2021;151(10):3205–13.
33. Schlanger LE, Bailey JL, Sands JM. Electrolytes in the aging. Adv Chronic Kidney Dis 2010;17(4):308–19.
34. Dahl WJ, Stewart ML. Position of the academy of nutrition and dietetics: health implications of dietary fiber. J Acad Nutr Diet 2015;115(11):1861–70.
35. Willis HJ, Thomas W, Willis DJ, et al. Feasibility of measuring gastric emptying time, with a wireless motility device, after subjects consume fiber-matched liquid and solid breakfasts. Appetite 2011;57(1):38–44.
36. Reynolds A, Mann J, Cummings J, et al. Carbohydrate quality and human health: a series of systematic reviews and meta-analyses. Lancet 2019;393(10170):434–45.
37. Nutrition Assistance Programs. Agencies could do more to help address the nutritional needs of older adults. In: Office USGA, ed2019.
38. In: Ross AC, Taylor CL, Yaktine AL, et al, eds. Dietary reference intakes for calcium and vitamin D. Washington, DC. 2011.

39. Meehan M, Penckofer S. The role of vitamin D in the aging adult. J Aging Gerontol 2014;2(2):60–71.
40. Roth DE, Abrams SA, Aloia J, et al. Global prevalence and disease burden of vitamin D deficiency: a roadmap for action in low- and middle-income countries. Ann N Y Acad Sci 2018;1430(1):44–79.
41. Balk EM, Adam GP, Langberg VN, et al. Global dietary calcium intake among adults: a systematic review. Osteoporos Int 2017;28(12):3315–24.
42. In: Dietary reference intakes for thiamin, riboflavin, niacin, vitamin B6, folate, vitamin B12, pantothenic acid, biotin, and choline. Washington, DC. 1998.
43. Pfisterer KJ, Sharratt MT, Heckman GG, et al. Vitamin B12 status in older adults living in Ontario long-term care homes: prevalence and incidence of deficiency with supplementation as a protective factor. Appl Physiol Nutr Metab 2016; 41(2):219–22.
44. Wong CW, Ip CY, Leung CP, et al. Vitamin B12 deficiency in the institutionalized elderly: a regional study. Exp Gerontol 2015;69:221–5.
45. Cavalcoli F, Zilli A, Conte D, et al. Micronutrient deficiencies in patients with chronic atrophic autoimmune gastritis: a review. World J Gastroenterol 2017; 23(4):563–72.
46. Weck MN, Stegmaier C, Rothenbacher D, et al. Epidemiology of chronic atrophic gastritis: population-based study among 9444 older adults from Germany. Aliment Pharmacol Ther 2007;26(6):879–87.
47. Iron MW-R. In: Ross ACCB, Cousins RJ, Tucker KL, et al, editors. Modern nutrition in health and disease. 11th edition. Baltimore (MD): Lippincott Williams & Wilkin; 2014. p. 176–88.
48. Fairweather-Tait SJ, Wawer AA, Gillings R, et al. Iron status in the elderly. Mech Ageing Dev 2014;136-137:22–8.
49. In: Dietary reference intakes for vitamin A, vitamin K, arsenic, boron, chromium, copper, iodine, iron, manganese, molybdenum, nickel, silicon, vanadium, and zinc. Washington, DC. 2001.
50. Vaudin A, Wambogo E, Moshfegh AJ, et al. Sodium and potassium intake, the sodium to potassium ratio, and associated characteristics in older adults, NHANES 2011-2016. J Acad Nutr Diet 2022;122(1):64–77.
51. Whelton PK. Sodium, potassium, blood pressure, and cardiovascular disease in humans. Curr Hypertens Rep 2014;16(8):465.
52. Dietary guidelines for Americans, 2020-2025. U.S. Department of Agriculture and Health and Human Services; 2020.
53. English LK, Ard JD, Bailey RL, et al. Evaluation of dietary patterns and all-cause mortality: a systematic review. JAMA Netw Open 2021;4(8):e2122277.
54. Lichtenstein AH, Appel LJ, Vadiveloo M, et al. Dietary Guidance to improve cardiovascular health: a scientific statement from the american heart association. Circulation 2021;144(23):e472–87.
55. Roberts SB, Silver RE, Das SK, et al. Healthy aging-nutrition matters: start early and screen often. Adv Nutr 2021;12(4):1438–48.
56. Lichtenstein AH, Rasmussen H, Yu WW, et al. Modified mypyramid for older adults. J Nutr 2008;138(1):5–11.
57. 2015-2020 Dietary Guidelines for Americans. U.S. Department of Health and Human Services and U.S. Department of Agriculture.; 2015.

Update on Nutrition in Diabetes Management

Andrew Reynolds, PhD*, Jim Mann, MD, PhD

KEYWORDS

- Diabetes management • Dietary recommendations • Evidence-based medicine

KEY POINTS

- Nutrition is a cornerstone of blood glucose control in diabetes management alongside physical activity, education, medication adherence, and regular check-ups.
- Although nutrition therapy may be prescribed in different ways (eg, advice regarding nutrients, foods, food groups, dietary patterns), key recommendations for people with diabetes are the same as those for the total population.
- All approaches encourage regular intakes of minimally processed whole grains, nuts, legumes, vegetables, and whole fruit, whereas minimizing the consumption of red and processed meat, added sugars, added sodium, refined grains, and ultraprocessed foods.

Before the introduction of insulin in the 1920s and oral hypoglycemic agents some 30 years later, advice to reduce carbohydrate intake was the only widely accepted therapeutic option for the management of diabetes.[1] Dietary advice for diabetes management has been less consistent since then, resulting in confusion and uncertainty among health professionals and people with diabetes.[2,3] This confusion is not helped by claims in the scientific literature and media that widely discrepant ways of eating offer unique benefits. As part of a move to counter such confusion, evidence-based dietary recommendations for people with diabetes have been issued in many countries.[4] These recommendations are principally supported by systematic reviews and meta analyses of trials in which dietary manipulations have been shown to improve glycemic control, or other cardiometabolic risk factors, and observational epidemiologic studies reporting on premature mortality and noncommunicable disease occurrence. Data derived from the general population complement the information available from studies of people with diabetes.

More recently, dietary guidelines have also provided an indication of the certainty of the available evidence, typically applying a known framework such as Grading of Recommendations, Assessment, Development and Evaluations (GRADE).[5] Certainty relates to the consistency in which an exposure (diet) changes a health outcome.

Department of Medicine, University of Otago, PO Box 56, Dunedin 9054, New Zealand
* Corresponding author.
E-mail address: andrew.reynolds@otago.ac.nz

Med Clin N Am 106 (2022) 865–879
https://doi.org/10.1016/j.mcna.2022.03.003
0025-7125/22/© 2022 Elsevier Inc. All rights reserved.

medical.theclinics.com

GRADE processes consider the risk of bias within a body of evidence to determine if the evidence is of high, moderate, low, or very-low certainty. Data from observational studies begin at low certainty and data from randomized controlled trials begin at high, given the inherent strengths or flaws of the study design. The body of evidence can then be either downgraded (eg, for highly inconsistent results between trials) or upgraded (visible dose response) in certainty. Assessing the certainty of evidence available enhances the transparency of the guideline development process and goes on to inform how a recommendation is worded.[6]Most recommendations made here are of moderate to high certainty, with the evidence profile provided in the references systematic reviews and meta analayses.

Nutrition therapy is considered alongside the other cornerstones of diabetes management: physical activity, education, medication adherence, and regular checkups (Fig. 1). Current dietary recommendations tend to be less rigid than those in the past and acknowledge that quality of life and needs of the individual and family must be considered. Health professionals should acknowledge the need for a balance between achieving optimal glycemic and other cardiometabolic risk factor control and the preferences and capacity of the patient. However, these considerations should not undermine the fact that dietary choice has the potential to profoundly improve or impair diabetes management. Key recommendations from this document are summarized in Table 1.

BODY WEIGHT
What Is New

- A range of low-energy diets is suitable for weight loss, provided they are acceptable to the patient and adhered to.
- Sustained weight loss of 10% to 15% body weight in those who are obese can achieve remission of type 2 diabetes.

Although genetic factors determine susceptibility,[7] the rapidly escalating rates of T2DM are largely explained by the almost worldwide increase in overweight and obesity.[8] Reducing excess adiposity substantially reduces the chances of those with prediabetes progressing to diabetes.[9] The Finnish Diabetes Prevention Study was the first published randomized controlled trial, which showed an approximately 60% reduction in risk of progression to T2DM in people with impaired glucose

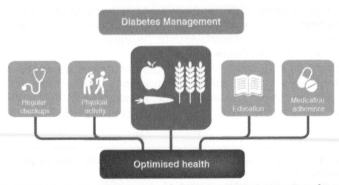

Fig. 1. Role of diet alongside other aspects of diabetes management. *Data from* Stephen J. D. O'Keefe, et al., Trypsin and splanchnic protein turnover during feeding and fasting in human subjects, American Journal of Physiology-Gastrointestinal and Liver Physiology 2006 290:2, G213-G221.

Table 1	
Key aspects of nutrition therapy for diabetes management	
Body weight	Achieve or maintain BMI of 18.5-25
	If overweight or obese, a reduced energy intake is essential for weight loss
	To achieve Type 2 diabetes mellitus (T2DM) remission, maintain a body weight reduction of 10%-15% if initial overweight or obese.
Carbohydrate	A wide range of carbohydrate intakes is acceptable provided saturated fat intakes do not exceed recommendations
	Carbohydrate sources should be high in fiber, such as minimally processed whole grains, vegetables, legumes, seeds, nuts, and whole fruits
	Added sugar intake should not exceed 10% total energy
Fat	Saturated and *trans*-unsaturated fat should comprise <10% and <1% total energy, respectively
	When reducing saturated and trans-fat, replacement should be with polyunsaturated or *cis*-monosaturated fats coming from seeds, nuts, and nontropical vegetable oils
	Reduction of total fat to <30% Total energy (TE) may facilitate weight loss
Protein	For most protein should provide 10%–20% total energy
	Total protein intake at lower end of normal range may be best for patients with established nephropathy
	Higher protein intakes (up to 30% TE) in those with diabetes and normal renal function may improve measures of glycemic control, blood pressure, and body weight
Micronutrients	Restrict salt to <6 g/d (<2.3 g sodium). Reduce further if hypertensive
Foods	Ensure food choices are for minimally processed foods, avoiding those that are ultraprocessed
Food groups	Choose wholegrain foods over refined grain products
Dietary patterns	A wide range of patterns are beneficial provided they are largely plant based (minimally processed whole grains, intact fruits and vegetables, and often also legumes and pulses) with fat sources that contain largely polyunsaturated or *cis*-monounsaturated fatty acids

tolerance advised to achieve modest weight loss (typically 5%–7% of initial body weight), compared with a control group.[10] Weight loss was achieved on a diet relatively low in total and saturated fat (less than 30% and 10% total energy, respectively) with whole grains, vegetables, and fruit providing most of the dietary carbohydrate while ensuring a dietary fiber intake of at least 15g per 1000 kcal. Benefits of similar dietary interventions (which included advice to undertake at least 30 minutes of physical activity of moderate intensity daily) were evident for 20 years or more after completion of the active intervention period.[11] Remarkably similar results were reported from the US Diabetes Prevention Project, which additionally found the dietary intervention to be more effective than treatment with metformin.[12]

Recent systematic reviews of randomized trials have clarified that even modest weight reduction in the overweight or obese improves insulin sensitivity, glycemic control, blood lipids, blood pressure, and other cardiovascular risk factors.[8] Weight loss may reduce or eliminate the need for hypoglycemic drug therapy in type 2 diabetes[13] and lead to a reduction of insulin dose and improved glycemic control in type 1 diabetes.[14] The reduced life expectancy of overweight people with diabetes is improved in those who lose weight.[15]

The key recommendation for people with T2DM or T1DM who are overweight (BMI >25 kg/m^2) or obese (BMI >30 kg/m^2) with central adiposity is that energy intake should be reduced so that the BMI moves toward the recommended range (18.5–

25 kg/m²). Recent systematic reviews of different weight loss diets in those with type 2 diabetes indicate that macronutrient distribution or dietary pattern followed are not important determinants of weight loss.[13] Rather, a range of reduced energy diets were identified as suitable for weight loss, provided they are acceptable to the patient. Low carbohydrate diets were no better than higher carbohydrate diets for weight loss,[16] with the macronutrient distribution having little impact on body weight compared with a reduction in energy intake.[13] More extreme energy reduction, such as with total diet replacement (providing 850 kcal/d) for 8 to 12 weeks led to an average 6.6 kg more weight loss compared with food-based low-energy diets.[13] Perhaps surprisingly, energy restriction beyond this (eg, very-low energy total meal replacement of 420–554 kcal/d) did not show greater weight reduction,[13] perhaps due to lower patient adherence to a stricter regimen. Increased energy expenditure through greater physical activity may also facilitate greater weight loss.

Appreciable sustained weight loss (10%–15% body weight) can achieve remission of type 2 diabetes, defined as HbA1c less than 48 mmol/mol after at least 2 months of all antidiabetic medication.[13] This has been demonstrated after bariatric surgery in people who are markedly obese.[17] More recently, based on the findings of a randomized controlled trial, The Diabetes Remission Clinical Trial (DIRECT), Lean and colleagues have shown that remission may also occur with weight loss of 15 kg or more achieved by initial use of low-energy total meal replacement of 12 weeks followed by reintroduction of solid food under the supervision of dietitians and a weight loss maintenance phase of 12 months.[18] Current evidence from this randomized controlled trial indicates the effects of such an intervention persist for at least 2 years.[19] Weight loss maintenance is particularly important as published case series and clinical observation suggest that diabetes recurs if weight loss is not sustained.

Alcohol may be a relevant source of energy in those who are overweight and may be associated with raised levels of blood pressure, increased triglycerides, and an increased risk of hypoglycemia, especially in insulin-treated individuals or those on some oral hypoglycemic agents. Although it is recommended that moderate use of alcohol (up to 10 g/d for women and 20 g/d for men) is acceptable for those with diabetes who choose to drink alcohol, further restrictions are recommended for some. Alcohol should be limited by those who are overweight, hypertensive, or hypertryglyceridemic. When alcohol is taken by those on insulin, it is important that it be taken with carbohydrate-containing food to avoid the risk of potentially profound and prolonged hypoglycemia. Abstention is advised for those with diabetes who are also pregnant or with a history of alcohol abuse, pancreatitis, hypertriglyceridemia, and advanced neuropathy.

CARBOHYDRATE
What Is New

- Quality of carbohydrate in the diet is more important than quantity.
- Dietary fiber content is a key measure of carbohydrate quality.

Debate continues regarding the optimal proportion of total energy that should be derived from dietary carbohydrate. Protagonists of low carbohydrate diets or very-low carbohydrate-ketogenic diets claim that such diets result in greater weight loss, improved glycemic control (typically reflected in lower levels of Hb A1c), and a more favorable lipid profile when compared with higher carbohydrate diets in people with T2DM. Systematic reviews and meta-analyses that attempt to synthesize existing knowledge are not always helpful given that there is no universal agreement regarding the definitions of "very low," "lower," and "low" carbohydrate intakes. Meta-analyses that have been undertaken indicate when low and balanced carbohydrate diets are compared head-to-head; there are no clinically significant long-term differences in glycemia, lipids, blood pressure, or weight control.[16,20–22] Pertinent to recommendations regarding optimal intakes of total carbohydrate are the observations from meta-analyses of cohort studies in the general population, which suggest that carbohydrate intakes of less than 40% or more than 70% total energy are associated with greater premature mortality than moderate carbohydrate intakes.[23–25]

Arguably of greater importance to nutrition recommendations than the proportion of total energy provided by carbohydrate is the quality of the carbohydrate consumed,[26] given carbohydrates range from simple sugar structures to large complex fibers.[1] Randomized controlled trials have shown that foods rich in dietary fiber such as whole grains and total dietary fiber regardless of source have the potential to improve glycemic control and improve cardiometabolic risk factors when compared with lower intakes.[26,27] Observational data provide strong support for translating these findings into nutrition recommendations.[26,27] One of the largest meta-analysis of prospective cohort studies to date indicates that higher intakes of dietary fiber are associated with appreciably reduced risks of developing type 2 diabetes.[26] In those with prediabetes, type 1, or type 2 diabetes cohorts, with higher intakes of dietary fiber have reduced premature mortality.[27] Benefits are apparent across the range of intakes but the data suggest that increasing fiber by 15g or to 35 g/d would contribute to the reduction of premature mortality in adults with diabetes.[26] These findings are consistent with trials showing benefits of dietary fiber on cardiometabolic risk factors and therefore serve as a reasonable target intake. Five or more servings per day of fiber-rich vegetables and fruit and 4 or more servings of legumes per week would help to ensure that these minimum requirements for fiber intake would be achieved provided most cereal-based foods were fiber-rich whole grains. The key carbohydrate recommendation for people with T2DM or T1DM is that a wide range of intakes is acceptable provided carbohydrate comes largely from minimally processed whole grains, vegetables, legumes, seeds, nuts, and whole fruits that are rich sources of fiber.

There has of late been rather less emphasis on the importance of restriction of dietary sugars than was the case previously. This is largely due to the fact that sugars have not been directly implicated as a cause of diabetes and because crossover trials in people with diabetes have shown that incorporating modest amounts (<50 g/d) of sucrose into diets of appropriate macronutrient composition and energy content, seems not to be associated with any measurable untoward clinical or metabolic effects.[28] However, high intakes of dietary sugars may be associated with weight gain in people with diabetes as in the case in the general population[29,30] and contribute to poor glycemic control[31] and deterioration of the dyslipidemia of the metabolic syndrome.[32] Therefore, it is advised that the intake of total free sugars should not exceed 10%TE as per the recommendation of the WHO for population at large,[33] although more restrictive advice concerning free sugars is appropriate for those needing to lose weight, those with poor glycemic control, and those with dyslipidemia (high triglycerides, low High denisty lipoprotein [HDL]).[33] Sugar-sweetened beverages should be avoided.

Several methods have been developed to describe the quality of carbohydrate in carbohydrate-containing foods beyond measures of constituents (eg, fiber, sugar). Glycemic index (GI) and glycemic load (GL) are the most widely used. GI is a standardized method for comparing the postprandial glycemic responses of carbohydrate-containing foods.[34] The metric indicates the postprandial glycemic response as a proportion of the response observed following a comparable oral glucose load. High (>70) or low (<40) GI values are likely to reflect carbohydrate quality; however, small differences may be of little relevance because there is considerable interindividual and intraindividual variations in glycemic response. GL is a similar metric but considers the amount of carbohydrate within the food.

Dietary GI or GL are different metrics that characterizes an individual's overall diet by a GI or GL value. Calculations are usually based on self-reported dietary intakes from food diaries or Food Frequency Questionnaires. Findings from systematic reviews of randomized controlled trials and prospective observation data from the general population do not indicate dietary GI or GL as useful predictors of premature mortality, heart disease or type 2 diabetes incidence, or change in cardiometabolic risk factors body weight, glycemia, blood lipids, or blood pressure.[26] However, recent meta-analysis of randomized trials focused on individuals with type 2 diabetes indicate lower dietary GI is useful in improving glycemic control.[35] If GI or GL is used as a guide to food choice, these foods also need to meet recommendations for fiber, sugars, protein, sodium, and saturated fat intakes.

DIETARY FAT
What Is New

- Replacement of Saturated fats (SFA) with Monounsaturated fats (MUFA) or Ployunsaturated fats (PUFA) improves lipid profile in those with diabetes.

Dietary fats are present in or added to many foods in the food supply and comprise around 30% of total energy intake in the United States.[36] Until recently the advice for people with diabetes has largely been based on data derived from the general population, to restrict saturated fat intake to less than 10% total energy.[37] High-saturated fat intakes have the potential to increase low-density lipoprotein (LDL) cholesterol concentrations and increase risk of cardiovascular disease.[38–40] Furthermore a high intake of saturated fatty acids increases resistance to the action of insulin,[41] and is therefore likely to increase the risk of developing type 2 diabetes. The striking relationships between saturated and trans-unsaturated fatty acids, and total and LDL cholesterol and Coronary Heart Disease (CHD) justify the recommendation to restrict intakes. All dietary trans-fat should be avoided as much as possible and kept less than 1% total energy.[42] Replacement of SFA with cis monounsaturated and polyunsaturated fatty acids-containing foods is associated with a reduction in LDL cholesterol levels, an improvement in several other cardiometabolic risk factors,[43] and reduction in CHD risk.[44]

Studies in people with diabetes confirm that these benefits initially observed in healthy populations also apply to those with the condition.[44] The key recommendation regarding fat for people with T2DM or T1DM is consume foods containing plant-based monounsaturated and polyunsaturated fats (seeds, nuts, avocado and fish with the use of by using nontropical vegetable oils) rather than saturated or trans-fats (meats, processed meats, butter, coconut products and palm oil).

Most guidelines do not specify an upper limit of intake for total fat. This permits a flexible approach to the selection of food choices and dietary patterns. However, given the energy density of fat, some restriction of total fat (to no more than 30% TE) may help to reduce energy intake and then body fat in those who are overweight and obese.

PROTEIN
What Is New

- For adults with type 2 diabetes but without nephropathy, higher protein intakes may reduce body weight, fasting blood glucose, and blood pressure.
- Higher intakes (up to 30% TE) are acceptable in the short term (up to 12 months) in those with normal renal function.

Protein intake in the United States is between 10% and 20% TE,[45] corresponding approximately to 0.8 to 1.3 g/kg body weight. This range seems appropriate for most people with diabetes. Intakes at the higher end of the range are acceptable for people with diabetes who do not have evidence of diabetic renal disease or nephropathy. More recent evidence synthesis involving trials of adults with type 2 diabetes without nephropathy indicate intake ranging between 15% and 20%TE may also help to maintain muscle mass and avoid sarcopenia in older people (aged 65 years or older).[46] Published guidelines for diabetes management do not directly consider the risk of high protein intake[47–49]; hence, more moderate intakes may be appropriate in the long term.

In patients with type 1 diabetes and evidence of established nephropathy, protein intakes should be at the lower,[50] corresponding to approximately 0.8 g/kg body weight/d. Such restriction may reduce the risk of end-stage renal failure or death when compared in randomized controlled trials, with more usual intakes (1.3 g/kg/d).[51] The evidence for appreciably reducing protein intake is less convincing for type 2 diabetes patients with established nephropathy or for type 1 or type 2 diabetes patients with microalbuminuria (incipient nephropathy). There is insufficient evidence comparing plant-based proteins with animal proteins to provide comment on this topic at present.

MICRONUTRIENTS

Foods naturally rich in minerals, vitamins, and dietary antioxidants are encouraged. Daily consumption of a range of vegetables, fruits, and whole grain breads and cereals should provide adequate intakes of vitamins and antioxidant nutrients. Given the tendency toward high levels of blood pressure in people with diabetes, restriction of salt intake to less than 6 g/d (2300 mg sodium) is advised,[52] with further restriction considered appropriate for those with elevated blood pressure levels. There is insufficient evidence to recommend the use of antioxidant supplements or preparations of other small compounds extracted from food in the management of diabetes.

FOOD AND FOOD GROUPS
What Is New

- Ultraprocessed foods are the main source of dietary energy in many countries, with emerging evidence indicating higher intakes associated with poor health outcomes.
- Processing of wholegrain foods beyond dehulling increases their postprandial blood response.
- Whole grains and refined grains should be considered as separate food groups.

There is no single food that is of particular benefit or detriment to those with diabetes. Foods advertised as being useful for people with diabetes ("diabetic" foods) are generally sucrose-free, but may nevertheless be high in fructose or other nutritive sweeteners, and sometimes saturated or trans-fat.

One trend of note within the food supply is the increased availability and intake of ultraprocessed foods. Ultraprocessed foods are "ready-to-consume and ready-to-heat formulations, made by combining substances derived from foods with cosmetic additives, typically through a series of industrial processes."[53] Recent estimates indicate Ultraprocessed foods (UPFs) are the main source of dietary energy in high income countries,[54] with low-middle income countries rapidly catching up.[55] Several methods to categorize the level of food processing now exist.[56] Observational data indicate greater total mortality, coronary heart disease, type 2 diabetes, obesity, and certain cancers in those reporting higher intakes of ultraprocessed foods.[57–65] Emerging data indicate UPF consumption differs between ethnicities and is greater in low-income and less educated groups,[66] suggesting a role in increasing health inequities.

Limited interventional data exist on the role of food processing in the management of diabetes. Recently published acute and short-term studies in adults with type 2 diabetes have shown that milling whole grains is associated with a greater glycemic response than consumption of less or unmilled whole grains.[67–69] A controlled feeding study of participants without diabetes has linked food processing to greater energy intakes.[70] Although additional confirmatory data are required, these emerging findings support the suggestion that dietary recommendations should promote foods that are minimally processed.

Intake of vegetables and fruit are universally recommended, given their low-energy density, micronutrient and fiber content, and lack of saturated fats or sodium.[1] Higher intake of vegetables and fruit in the population at large are associated with reduced premature mortality and noncommunicable disease occurrence[71] as they would be in those with diabetes. Concerns about root vegetable intake, such as potatoes, seems to relate more to the cooking method than the vegetable itself, with intake of boiled and roasted potato largely unrelated to poor health outcomes.[72] Whole fruit intake has been proven beneficial, however food processing such as drying and juicing will likely cause higher levels of intake than if consuming the intact fruit. Grain foods are often promoted, with a strong focus on whole grains due to the considerable benefits associated with their intake[26,27] compared with refined grains. Most grain foods purchased in America are refined rather than whole grain,[73] presenting an opportunity for clear dietary messages toward healthier intakes. Recommendations for both dairy and "protein based" food groups focus on the low-fat options within these food groups such as milk and yoghurt with some cheese for dairy, or fish, eggs, legumes, tofu, nuts and seeds, or very lean meats for protein foods.

DIETARY PATTERNS
What Is New

- A variety of dietary patterns that have common attributes are appropriate for people with diabetes.
- No single dietary pattern is best for diabetes management.

Recent evidence synthesis of data from randomized trials indicate that blood glucose control, weight loss, and weight maintenance may be achieved by several different dietary patterns (eg, Mediterranean,[74,75] Nordic,[76] Vegetarian,[77,78] Dietary approaches to stop hypertension (DASH[79]) in which carbohydrate is predominantly derived from minimally processed grains, intact fruits and vegetables and often also legumes and pulses, while fat sources are those which contain largely polyunsaturated or cis-monounsaturated fatty acids. A key point regarding dietary patterns is that no one pattern is superior, many share common traits and can therefore be determined by patient preference. High fat and Paleo dietary patterns are not recommended for long-term use because there is no evidence that they are safe or beneficial when used for prolonged periods. There have been dramatic increases in diabetes and obesity prevalence associated either with migration or with a rapid change from a traditional (non-Western) lifestyle to increased consumption of energy-dense processed foods, high in fats and sugars, and reduced levels of physical activity. These patterns (eg, a Western dietary pattern) relate to the increased availability of ultraprocessed foods, as discussed above. The American Pima Indians, Polynesians, and

Melanesians in the South Pacific, Australian Aboriginals, and Asian Indian migrants to the United Kingdom and other countries are examples of populations in which the process of rapid acculturation has led to diabetes prevalence rates far higher than those observed in European populations.[80]

NUTRITION WITHIN THE LIFESTYLE
What Is New

- Changing the food environment and societal factors are key facilitators to dietary change.
- The environmental sustainability of dietary choices is important and provides a new angle to promote minimally processed plant-based diets.

Individual adherence to dietary advice is improved if the advice is understood by the whole family and is of potential benefit to all members. In view of the strong genetic component to type 2 diabetes, the evidence that lifestyle changes reduce the risk of developing the condition, and that the dietary principles are similar to those recommended for the general population, it seems reasonable to recommend that foods and meals that are suitable for people with diabetes are appropriate for their families as well. Adoption of public health measures aimed at facilitating healthy food choices such as ensuring the availability of appropriate foods at reasonable cost are necessary, whereas increasing the cost of certain foods (eg, sugary drinks) may prove beneficial provided any revenue accrued from such taxation is committed back into public health initiatives.

An emerging field of research relating to food choice and the consequences of our choices is the environmental sustainability of food production. Food production accounts for 26% of greenhouse gas emissions globally, with beef the largest food source of emissions.[81] Current global eating patterns do not meet environmental targets for greenhouse gas emissions, freshwater use, cropland use, and fertilizer application[82] with current dietary intake transitioning globally toward greater meat intake.[83] Climate change, of which food production contributes considerably, is now this century's greatest global health threat.[84] The evidence available in this area indicates that movement away from animal source foods toward a greater diversified plant-based intake would increase likeliness of meeting environmental targets,[85] and reduce human-made pressure on the environment.[86]

SUMMARY

Health professionals may not often have the training or the time to support people with diabetes translate the dietary recommendations described here into practice. However, nutrition is a cornerstone of diabetes management and should be regarded as fundamental to achieving blood glucose control. More recent evidence on topics such as body weight and dietary patterns indicate flexibility in what can be recommended, which enables patient preference and may aid adherence. Importantly, a healthy diet for those with diabetes is also appropriate to recommend for their families and the general population, increasing the relevance of understanding and applying current evidence-based dietary guidelines.

CLINICS CARE POINTS

- Inform patients that dietary advice is given to reduce risk of disease and improve quality of life.

- Given the misinformation available, ensure advice to patients is reflective of current evidence-based recommendations.
- Dietary advice should be as practical as possible, formulated in discussion with the patient to be achievable for them and their family.
- Dietary advice is an ongoing component of patient care.

DISCLOSURE OF INTEREST

J. Mann is funded by the Healthier Lives National Science Challenge. A. Reynolds is funded by the National Heart Foundation of New Zealand. Both authors are members of the Edgar Diabetes and Obesity Research Center. The authors report no other relationships or activities that could seem to have influenced the submitted article.

REFERENCES

1. Truswell S, Mann J. Essentials of human nutrition. Oxford: Oxford University Press; 2017.
2. Mozaffarian D. Dietary and policy priorities to reduce the global crises of obesity and diabetes. Nat Food 2020;1(1):38–50.
3. Booth AO, Lowis C, Dean M, Hunter SJ, McKinley MC. Diet and physical activity in the self-management of type 2 diabetes: barriers and facilitators identified by patients and health professionals. Prim Health Care Res Development 2013; 14(3):293–306.
4. Dyson P, Twenefour D, Breen C, et al. Diabetes UK evidence-based nutrition guidelines for the prevention and management of diabetes. Diabetic Med 2018;35(5):541–7.
5. Guyatt GH, Oxman AD, Vist GE, et al. GRADE: an emerging consensus on rating quality of evidence and strength of recommendations. BMJ 2008;336(7650):924.
6. Alonso-Coello P, Oxman AD, Moberg J, et al. GRADE Evidence to Decision (EtD) frameworks: a systematic and transparent approach to making well informed healthcare choices. 2: Clinical practice guidelines. bmj 2016;353:i2089.
7. Tuomi T, Santoro N, Caprio S, Cai M, Weng J, Groop L. The many faces of diabetes: a disease with increasing heterogeneity. The Lancet 2014;383(9922): 1084–94.
8. Apovian CM, Okemah J, O'Neil PM. Body weight considerations in the management of type 2 diabetes. Adv Ther 2019;36(1):44–58.
9. Fonseca VA. Identification and Treatment of Prediabetes to Prevent Progression to Type 2 Diabetes. Clin Cornerstone 2008;9(2):51–61.
10. Tuomilehto J, Lindström J, Eriksson JG, et al. Prevention of type 2 diabetes mellitus by changes in lifestyle among subjects with impaired glucose tolerance. New Engl J Med 2001;344(18):1343–50.
11. Li G, Zhang P, Wang J, et al. Cardiovascular mortality, all-cause mortality, and diabetes incidence after lifestyle intervention for people with impaired glucose tolerance in the Da Qing Diabetes Prevention Study: a 23-year follow-up study. Lancet Diabetes Endocrinol 2014;2(6):474–80.
12. Knowler WC, Barrett-Connor E, Fowler SE, et al. Reduction in the incidence of type 2 diabetes with lifestyle intervention or metformin. N Engl J Med 2002;346: 393–403. https://doi.org/10.1056/NEJMoa012512.
13. Churuangsuk C, Hall J, Reynolds A. Diets for weight management in adults with type 2 diabetes: an umbrella review of published meta-analyses and systematic

review of trials of diets for diabetes remission. Diabetologia 2022;65(1):14–36. https://doi.org/10.1007/s00125-021-05577-2.

14. Polsky S, Ellis SL. Obesity, insulin resistance, and type 1 diabetes mellitus. Curr Opin Endocrinol Diabetes Obes 2015;22(4):277–82.

15. Williamson DF, Thompson TJ, Thun M, Flanders D, Pamuk E, Byers T. Intentional weight loss and mortality among overweight individuals with diabetes. Diabetes care 2000;23(10):1499–504.

16. Naude CE, Brand A, Schoonees A, Nguyen KA, Chaplin M, Volmink J. Low-carbohydrate versus balanced-carbohydrate diets for reducing weight and cardiovascular risk. Cochrane Database Syst Rev 2022;1(1):Cd013334.

17. Mingrone G, Panunzi S, De Gaetano A, et al. Bariatric surgery versus conventional medical therapy for type 2 diabetes. New Engl J Med 2012;366(17): 1577–85.

18. Lean ME, Leslie WS, Barnes AC, et al. Primary care-led weight management for remission of type 2 diabetes (DiRECT): an open-label, cluster-randomised trial. The Lancet 2018;391(10120):541–51.

19. Lean ME, Leslie WS, Barnes AC, et al. Durability of a primary care-led weight-management intervention for remission of type 2 diabetes: 2-year results of the DiRECT open-label, cluster-randomised trial. Lancet Diabetes Endocrinol 2019; 7(5):344–55.

20. Korsmo-Haugen HK, Brurberg KG, Mann J, Aas AM. Carbohydrate quantity in the dietary management of type 2 diabetes: a systematic review and meta-analysis. Diabetes Obes Metab 2019;21(1):15–27.

21. Snorgaard O, Poulsen GM, Andersen HK, Astrup A. Systematic review and meta-analysis of dietary carbohydrate restriction in patients with type 2 diabetes. BMJ Open Diabetes Res Care 2017;5(1).

22. Sainsbury E, Kizirian NV, Partridge SR, Gill T, Colagiuri S, Gibson AA. Effect of dietary carbohydrate restriction on glycemic control in adults with diabetes: a systematic review and meta-analysis. Diabetes Res Clin Pract 2018;139:239–52.

23. Noto H, Goto A, Tsujimoto T, Noda M. Low-carbohydrate diets and all-cause mortality: a systematic review and meta-analysis of observational studies. PLoS One 2013;8(1):e55030.

24. Seidelmann SB, Claggett B, Cheng S, et al. Dietary carbohydrate intake and mortality: a prospective cohort study and meta-analysis. The Lancet Public Health 2018;3(9):e419–28.

25. Mazidi M, Katsiki N, Mikhailidis DP, et al. Lower carbohydrate diets and all-cause and cause-specific mortality: a population-based cohort study and pooling of prospective studies. Eur Heart J 2019;40(34):2870–9.

26. Reynolds A, Mann J, Cummings J, Winter N, Mete E, Te Morenga L. Carbohydrate quality and human health: a series of systematic reviews and meta-analyses. The Lancet 2019;393(10170):434–45.

27. Reynolds AN, Akerman AP, Mann J. Dietary fibre and whole grains in diabetes management: systematic review and meta-analyses. PLoS Med 2020;17(3): e1003053.

28. Peterson D, Lambert J, Gerring S, et al. Sucrose in the diet of diabetic patients—just another carbohydrate? Diabetologia 1986;29(4):216–20.

29. World Health Organization. Sugars intake for adults and children: guideline. 2015. Ref Type: Report.Geneva (Switzerland): 2017.

30. Sievenpiper JL, de Souza RJ, Mirrahimi A, et al. Effect of fructose on body weight in controlled feeding trials: a systematic review and meta-analysis. Ann Intern Med 2012;156(4):291–304.

31. Choo VL, Viguiliouk E, Mejia SB, et al. Food sources of fructose-containing sugars and glycaemic control: systematic review and meta-analysis of controlled intervention studies. bmj 2018;363:k4644.
32. Semnani-Azad Z, Khan TA, Mejia SB, et al. Association of major food sources of fructose-containing sugars with incident metabolic syndrome: a systematic review and meta-analysis. JAMA Netw Open 2020;3(7):e209993.
33. World Health Organization. Guideline: sugars intake for adults and children. Geneva: World Health Organization; 2015.
34. International Organization for Standardization. Food products - determination of the glycaemic index (GI) and recommendation for food classification 26642-2010. Geneva: ISO; 2010.
35. Chiavaroli L, Lee D, Ahmed A, et al. Effect of low glycaemic index or load dietary patterns on glycaemic control and cardiometabolic risk factors in diabetes: systematic review and meta-analysis of randomised controlled trials. BMJ 2021;374: n1651.
36. Shan Z, Rehm CD, Rogers G, et al. Trends in Dietary Carbohydrate, Protein, and Fat Intake and Diet Quality Among US Adults, 1999-2016. JAMA 2019;322(12): 1178–87.
37. World Health Organization. Draft guidelines on saturated fatty acid and trans-fatty acid intake for adults and children. Geneva (Switzerland): World Health Organization; 2018. p. 103.
38. Mensink RP. Effects of saturated fatty acids on serum lipids and lipoproteins: a systematic review and regression analysis. Geneva: WHO Library Cataloguing-in-Publication Data; 2016.
39. Silverman MG, Ference BA, Im K, et al. Association Between Lowering LDL-C and cardiovascular risk reduction among different therapeutic interventions: a systematic review and meta-analysis. JAMA 2016;316(12):1289–97.
40. Ference BA, Ginsberg HN, Graham I, et al. Low-density lipoproteins cause atherosclerotic cardiovascular disease. 1. Evidence from genetic, epidemiologic, and clinical studies. A consensus statement from the European Atherosclerosis Society Consensus Panel. Eur Heart J 2017;38(32):2459–72.
41. Imamura F, Micha R, Wu JH, et al. Effects of saturated fat, polyunsaturated fat, monounsaturated fat, and carbohydrate on glucose-insulin homeostasis: a systematic review and meta-analysis of randomised controlled feeding trials. PLoS Med 2016;13(7):e1002087.
42. De Souza RJ, Mente A, Maroleanu A, et al. Intake of saturated and trans unsaturated fatty acids and risk of all cause mortality, cardiovascular disease, and type 2 diabetes: systematic review and meta-analysis of observational studies. BMJ 2015;351:h3978.
43. Mensink PRP. World Health Organization report: Effects of saturated fatty acids on serum lipids and lipoproteins: a systematic review and regression analysis. 2016.
44. Schwab U, Reynolds AN, Sallinen T. Dietary fat intakes and cardiovascular disease risk in adults with type 2 diabetes: a systematic review and meta-analysis. Eur J Nutr 2021;60(6):3355–63. https://doi.org/10.1007/s00394-021-02507-1.
45. Hoy K, Clemens J, Moshfegh A. Estimated Protein Intake from Animal and Plant Foods by US Adults, What We Eat in America, NHANES, 2015–2016. Curr Dev Nutr 2021;5(Supplement_2):133.
46. Pfeiffer AFH, Pedersen E, Schwab U, et al. The effects of different quantities and qualities of protein intake in people with diabetes mellitus. Nutrients 2020; 12(2):365.

47. Dworatzek PD, Arcudi K, Gougeon R, Husein N, Sievenpiper JL, Williams SL. Nutrition therapy. Can J Diabetes 2013;37:S45–55.
48. American Diabetes Association Professional Practice Committee. 8. Obesity and Weight Management for the Prevention and Treatment of Type 2 Diabetes: Standards of Medical Care in Diabetes—2022. Diabetes Care 2021; 45(Supplement_1):S113–24.
49. Diabetes UK. Evidence-based nutrition guidelines for the prevention and management of diabetes. London (UK): Diabetes UK; 2011.
50. Papadopoulou-Marketou N, Chrousos GP, Kanaka-Gantenbein C. Diabetic nephropathy in type 1 diabetes: a review of early natural history, pathogenesis, and diagnosis. Diabetes/Metabolism Res Rev 2017;33(2):e2841.
51. Robertson LM, Waugh N, Robertson A. Protein restriction for diabetic renal disease. Cochrane Database Syst Rev 2007;(4):CD002181.
52. World Health Organization. Guideline: sodium intake for adults and children. Geneva: World Health Organization; 2012.
53. Monteiro CA. Nutrition and health. The issue is not food, nor nutrients, so much as processing. Public Health Nutrition 2009;12(5):729–31.
54. Monteiro CA, Cannon G, Lawrence M, Costa Louzada Md, Pereira Machado P. Ultra-processed foods, diet quality, and health using the NOVA classification system. Rome: FAO; 2019. p. 48.
55. Scott P. Global panel on agriculture and food systems for nutrition: food systems and diets: facing the challenges of the 21st century. Springer; 2017.
56. Monteiro CA, Cannon G, Lawrence M, Costa Louzada Md, Pereira Machado P. Ultra-processed foods, diet quality, and health using the NOVA classification system. Rome (Italy): FAO; 2019.
57. Srour B, Fezeu LK, Kesse-Guyot E, et al. Ultra-processed food intake and risk of cardiovascular disease: prospective cohort study (NutriNet-Santé). BMJ 2019;365.
58. Narula N, Wong EC, Dehghan M, et al. Association of ultra-processed food intake with risk of inflammatory bowel disease: prospective cohort study. BMJ 2021;374: n1554.
59. Ivancovsky-Wajcman D, Fliss-Isakov N, Webb M, et al. Ultra-processed food is associated with features of metabolic syndrome and non-alcoholic fatty liver disease. Liver Int 2021;41(11):2635–45.
60. Rico-Campà A, Martínez-González MA, Alvarez-Alvarez I, et al. Association between consumption of ultra-processed foods and all cause mortality: SUN prospective cohort study. BMJ 2019;365:l1949.
61. Canella DS, Levy RB, Martins APB, et al. Ultra-processed food products and obesity in Brazilian households (2008–2009). PLoS One 2014;9(3):e92752.
62. Monteiro CA, Moubarac J-C, Levy RB, Canella DS, da Costa Louzada ML, Cannon G. Household availability of ultra-processed foods and obesity in nineteen European countries. Public Health Nutr 2018;21(1):18–26.
63. Fiolet T, Srour B, Sellem L, et al. Consumption of ultra-processed foods and cancer risk: results from NutriNet-Santé prospective cohort. BMJ 2018;360:k322.
64. Chen X, Zhang Z, Yang H, et al. Consumption of ultra-processed foods and health outcomes: a systematic review of epidemiological studies. Nutr J 2020; 19(1):1–10.
65. Kim H, Hu EA, Rebholz CM. Ultra-processed food intake and mortality in the USA: results from the Third National Health and Nutrition Examination Survey (NHANES III, 1988–1994). Public Health Nutr 2019;22(10):1777–85.

66. Baraldi LG, Martinez Steele E, Canella DS, Monteiro CA. Consumption of ultra-processed foods and associated sociodemographic factors in the USA between 2007 and 2012: evidence from a nationally representative cross-sectional study. BMJ Open 2018;8(3):e020574.

67. Reynolds AN, Mann J, Elbalshy M, et al. Wholegrain particle size influences post-prandial glycemia in type 2 diabetes: a randomized crossover study comparing four wholegrain breads. Diabetes Care 2020;43(2):476–9.

68. Reynolds AN, Mann JI, Elbalshy M. Wholegrain particle size influences postprandial glycaemia in type 2 diabetes: a randomised crossover study comparing four wholegrain breads. Diabetes Care 2020;43(2):476–9. https://doi.org/10.2337/dc19-1466.

69. Elbalshy MM, Reynolds AN, Mete E, et al. Gelatinisation and milling whole-wheat increases postprandial blood glucose: randomised crossover study of adults with type 2 diabetes. Diabetologia 2021;64(6):1385–8.

70. Hall KD, Ayuketah A, Brychta R, et al. Ultra-processed diets cause excess calorie intake and weight gain: an inpatient randomized controlled trial of ad libitum food intake. Cell Metab 2019;30(1):67–77.e3.

71. Aune D, Giovannucci E, Boffetta P, et al. Fruit and vegetable intake and the risk of cardiovascular disease, total cancer and all-cause mortality—a systematic review and dose-response meta-analysis of prospective studies. Int J Epidemiol 2017; 46(3):1029–56.

72. Schwingshackl L, Schwedhelm C, Hoffmann G, Boeing H. Potatoes and risk of chronic disease: A systematic review and dose–response meta-analysis. Eur J Nutr 2019;58(6):2243–51.

73. Dunford EK, Miles DR, Popkin B, Ng SW. Whole Grain and Refined Grains: An Examination of US Household Grocery Store Purchases. J Nutr 2021;152(2):550–8.

74. Esposito K, Maiorino MI, Bellastella G, Chiodini P, Panagiotakos D, Giugliano D. A journey into a Mediterranean diet and type 2 diabetes: a systematic review with meta-analyses. BMJ open 2015;5(8):e008222.

75. Díaz-López A, Babio N, Martínez-González MA, et al. Mediterranean diet, retinopathy, nephropathy, and microvascular diabetes complications: a post hoc analysis of a randomized trial. Diabetes care 2015;38(11):2134–41.

76. Adamsson V, Reumark A, Fredriksson IB, et al. Effects of a healthy Nordic diet on cardiovascular risk factors in hypercholesterolaemic subjects: a randomized controlled trial (NORDIET). J Intern Med 2011;269(2):150–9.

77. Glenn AJ, Lo K, Jenkins DJ, et al. Relationship Between a Plant-Based Dietary Portfolio and Risk of Cardiovascular Disease: Findings From the Women's Health Initiative Prospective Cohort Study. J Am Heart Assoc 2021;10(16):e021515.

78. Viguiliouk E, Kendall CW, Kahleová H, et al. Effect of vegetarian dietary patterns on cardiometabolic risk factors in diabetes: a systematic review and meta-analysis of randomized controlled trials. Clin Nutr 2019;38(3):1133–45.

79. Chiavaroli L, Viguiliouk E, Nishi SK, et al. DASH dietary pattern and cardiometabolic outcomes: an umbrella review of systematic reviews and meta-analyses. Nutrients 2019;11(2):338.

80. Williams DE, Knowler WC, Smith CJ, et al. The effect of Indian or Anglo dietary preference on the incidence of diabetes in Pima Indians. Diabetes care 2001; 24(5):811–6.

81. Poore J, Nemecek T. Reducing food's environmental impacts through producers and consumers. Science 2018;360(6392):987–92.

82. Springmann M, Spajic L, Clark MA, et al. The healthiness and sustainability of national and global food based dietary guidelines: modelling study. BMJ 2020;370: m2322.
83. Baker P, Machado P, Santos T, et al. Ultra-processed foods and the nutrition transition: Global, regional and national trends, food systems transformations and political economy drivers. Obes Rev 2020;21(12):e13126.
84. IPCC. Climate change 2014: synthesis report. Geneva (Switzerland): Intergovernmental Panel on Climate Change; 2014. ISBN 978-92-9169-143-2.
85. Clark MA, Springmann M, Hill J, Tilman D. Multiple health and environmental impacts of foods. Proc Natl Acad Sci 2019;116(46):23357–62.
86. Willett W, Rockström J, Loken B, et al. Food in the Anthropocene: the EAT–Lancet Commission on healthy diets from sustainable food systems. Lancet 2019; 393(10170):447–92.

Dietary Supplements – The Wild West of Good, Bad, and a Whole Lotta Ugly

Dónal O'Mathúna, BSc(Pharm), MA, PhD[a],*, Walter L. Larimore, MD[b]

KEYWORDS

- Dietary supplements • Natural medicines • Herbal remedies • Herbs vitamins
- Evidence • Advertising • Quality • Effectiveness • Safety • Cannabidiol • CBD
- Vitamin C

KEY POINTS

- Dietary supplements, herbal remedies, and vitamins (natural medicines) remain extremely popular with consumers.
- Evidence for the effectiveness, safety, and quality of many natural medicines is often lacking.
- Consumers often have both inaccurate beliefs and incomplete knowledge about natural medicines. For example, most believe "natural" means "safe."
- Regulation of and advertising of natural medications in the United States urgently needs revision to better protect public health.
- Clinicians and consumers need independent and trustworthy information about natural medicines along with independent laboratory testing of products identifying those inaccurately labeled or contaminated.

INTRODUCTION

The market for herbal remedies, dietary supplements, and vitamins (what are collectively called "natural medicines") continues to grow. For decades now, the interest in and purchasing of these products has not decreased. But neither have the concerns that we have been writing about for more than 20 years. Foremost among these is the myth that just because something is "natural," it must be safe.[1] The natural world contains many poisonous and dangerous things. Just because it's "natural" or has "natural" on the label, does not make something safe, and it also doesn't necessarily mean it will do any good.

[a] College of Nursing, Helene Fuld Health Trust National Institute for Evidence-based Practice in Nursing and Healthcare, The Ohio State University, Columbus, OH 43210, USA; [b] UCHealth Occupational Medicine Clinic, 13445 Voyager Pkwy, Colorado Springs, CO 80921, USA
* Corresponding author.
E-mail address: omathuna.6@osu.edu

Med Clin N Am 106 (2022) 881–898
https://doi.org/10.1016/j.mcna.2022.03.004
0025-7125/22/© 2022 Elsevier Inc. All rights reserved.

medical.theclinics.com

Questions that health professionals and their patients should all ask before recommending or taking *any* remedy or treatment include: What's the evidence that this works? If it works, will it work for my condition? What sorts of side effects might it have? Was it manufactured to the highest possible standards? Was it tested to make sure that what's on the label is in the bottle? And does it contain anything it shouldn't have in it?

A MULTI-BILLION DOLLAR INDUSTRY

Natural medicines are trendy across most of the developed world. According to a 2019 report, the global natural medicines market was valued at about $140 billion US dollars (USD) in 2018 and could reach over $216 billion USD by the year 2026, at a compound annual growth rate (CAGR) of 5.5%.[2] Another report estimated that the global dietary supplements market is expected to reach over $220 billion USD in 2022 while growing at a CAGR of 8.8%.[3]

Unfortunately, much of the advertising for these products is inaccurate, with the marketing claims far exceeding scientific data on safety and effectiveness. In a systematic review for the lay public, one of us (WL) evaluated about 1300 natural medicines or lifestyle interventions for about 550 conditions or indications. Two-thirds did not have evidence of safety or effectiveness—not only being a waste of time and money but in some cases even dangerous **(Table 1)**.[4]

INCREASING POPULARITY

Our best-selling books on alternative medicine and natural medicines[5,6] did very well with the public because the use of natural medications was hugely popular. It still is is, being approximately a $30 billion industry in the US, with over 90,000 products on the market in 2018.[7] In 2020, *Natural Medicines*™ listed over 185,000 products in the US and Canada.[8] Four out of five Americans regularly take a natural medicine.

A 2021 consumer survey by the Council for Responsible Nutrition (CRN) announced, "Supplement usage among Americans has steadily increased in the more than twenty years CRN has conducted the survey," adding, "With 80% of Americans now using supplements, these products are now mainstream and broadly accepted by the American public. Just as important, 79% of Americans believe the dietary

Table 1
Evidence available on the safety and effectiveness of 1300 natural interventions or medicines

~1300 Natural Medicines or Interventions Evaluated for		~550 Conditions/Indications	
★★★★★	83	6%	150	11%
★★★★	67	5%		
★★★	88	7%	269	22%
★★	69	5%		
★	103	10%		
☹	888	67%	888	67%

★★★★★ Effective and Likely Safe

★★★★ Likely Effective and Likely Safe

★★★ Effective and Possibly Safe

★★ Likely Effective and Possibly Safe OR Possibly Effective and Possibly Safe
★ Possibly Effective and Possibly Safe
☹ Insufficient Evidence, Possibly Ineffective, Possibly Unsafe, Ineffective, OR Unsafe

supplement industry is trustworthy, a jump of 5 percentage points from 2020." According to CRN, "50% of supplement users report a change to their supplement routine since the COVID-19 pandemic started, and 55% of those who reported a change indicated that it included adding new supplements to their existing routine."[9]

A 2019 national survey reported 86% of Americans took natural medicines, especially vitamins and dietary supplements[10] – with 48% of adults taking vitamins and 39% taking minerals—most to "maintain health and prevent disease."[11] Another national survey showed that 52% of US adults reported the use of at least 1 natural medicine a day[7] while 10% reported using at least 4 such products daily.[7] Although these percentages vary from source to source, depending upon who and how they surveyed, the point is that natural medicines are *very* popular.

WHAT PEOPLE ARE USING AND WHY?

What are the top reasons people provide for taking supplements? It varies by age group, but some themes run across the generations (**Table 2**).[12]

What are the most popular natural medicines? Different surveys give different pictures, but some similar patterns are visible. ConsumerLab, in its "2022 Survey of Vitamins & Supplement Users,"[13] reported on the responses of 8049 US adult subscribers (with over 80.6% taking at least 4 different supplements daily). Among the top 50 supplements, only 8 declined in popularity, while 42 showed an increase (**Table 3**).

In contrast, a CRN survey of 2006 adults in the US, of whom 1529 (76%) considered themselves supplement users, reported different findings (**Table 4**).[12]

Again, the disparate results reflect different populations surveyed and the use of different survey tools.

CONSUMERS BELIEVE NATURAL MEDICINES ARE SAFE, HEALTHY, AND EFFECTIVE

The Nation Center for Complementary and Integrative Health (NCCIH) writes, "A lot of people believe that when it comes to medicine, 'natural' is better, healthier, and safer than 'unnatural' or synthetic drugs." They add, "Some people also believe that 'natural' products are safe because they believe these medicines are free of chemicals."[14] Around the world, people seem sold on the marketing claims that these products will allow them to avoid the "toxic" drugs foisted upon them by "the evils of Big Pharma" that "seeks enormous profits over the health and well-being of the humans it serves."[15]

An article in *Science-Based Medicine* adds, "Supplements are marketed as safe, natural, and effective, and there is no question that messaging has been effective."[16] CRN states, "85% of Americans are confident in the safety and quality of supplements

Table 2		
Top reasons why people take supplements by age groups		
18–34 y	**35–54 y**	**55+ y**
Overall Wellness (42%)	Overall Wellness (47%)	Overall Wellness (49%)
Energy (37%)	Energy (33%)	Fill Nutrient Gaps (33%)
Hair, Skin, Nails (28%)	Fill Nutrient Gaps (32%)	Bone Health (31%)
Immune Health (25%)	Immune Health (31%)	Heart Health (29%)
Fill Nutrient Gaps (22%)	Hair, Skin, Nails (23%)	Healthy Aging (28%)
Weight Management (21%)	Digestive Health (21%)	Joint Health (23%)

Table 3
Top supplements taken by consumers (ConsumerLab.com survey)

1. Vitamin D	Vitamin D (−0.4 pts) remained the most popular supplement, purchased by 72.6% of respondents.
2. Magnesium	With a continued rise in popularity, magnesium secured its place as the second most popular supplement and is used by 51.8% of respondents.
3. Fish oil	Was surpassed by magnesium for third place.
4. CoQ10:	Remained in fourth place.
5. Multivitamins	43.3% of respondents, +1.0 pts
6. Vitamin C (including Rose Hips)	41.9%, −0.1 pts
7. Probiotic (eg, Acidophilus, Lactobacillus)	38.7%, +2.3 pts
8. Zinc	36.9%, +1.2 pts
9. Curcumin/Turmeric (as Supplement)	35.9%, +2.3 pts
10. Vitamin B12 (Cobalamin)	33.3%, +4.0 pts

Data from ConsumerLab.com survey.

overall—and, unsurprisingly, in vitamins and minerals especially, which received an 88% confidence response." Additionally, CRN added, "76% of Americans perceive the dietary supplement industry as being trustworthy."[12]

Unfortunately, false advertising, inflated claims, poor manufacturing practices, inaccurate labeling, and contaminated products are far more common than most health professionals and consumers suspect.

NATURAL MEDICINES ARE PROBLEMATIC

JoAnn Manson, MD, chief of the Division of Preventive Medicine at Brigham and Women's Hospital in Boston, states, "Most supplements on the market are not tested for either efficacy or safety."[17] In contrast with "pharmaceuticals, which undergo extensive testing to prove they're effective and safe before they can be sold, dietary supplements can be sold without proof of effectiveness or safety. Moreover, supplement makers can claim their products enhance health, despite a dearth of evidence in most cases."[18] A 2018 editorial in the Journal of the American Medical Association (JAMA) added, "Clinicians and patients should also be aware that the US Food and Drug Administration is not authorized to review dietary supplements for safety and efficacy prior to marketing."[19]

Table 4
Top supplements taken by consumers (CRN survey)

1. Multivitamins	58%
2. Vitamin D	31%
3. Vitamin C	28%
4. Protein	21%
5. Calcium	20%
6. Vitamin B or B complex	20%
7. Omega 3 fatty acids or fish oil	16%

Data from CRN survey.

ILLEGAL CLAIMS ABOUND

Natural Medicines explains, "Most dietary supplements cannot legally claim to treat, cure, or prevent a disease. Doing so makes them legally unapproved drugs."[20] Unfortunately, the FDA and the Federal Trade Commission (FTC) often must issue warning letters to companies because of "advertisements and labels touting the supplements' ability to treat or cure Alzheimer's, cancer, and myriad other diseases. The warning letters specifically call out the manufacturers for making unapproved drug claims and deceptive statements."[21] *Natural Medicines* explains that "many supplement companies bank on the ignorance of consumers and continue to skate this line. It can sway those with serious medical conditions away from using proven therapies."[20]

MANUFACTURING, LABELING, AND CONTAMINATION ISSUES REMAIN COMMON

In 2010 testimony before the US Congress, Tod Cooperman, MD, the President and Founder of ConsumerLab.com, cited common problems with natural medicines sold in America (**Box 1**).[22]

Unfortunately, the situation has not improved greatly. In early 2020, ConsumerLab reported that about one in 5 supplements in the US and Canada that they tested did not meet one or more quality parameters. This is true even though ConsumerLab's testing tends to focus on the more popular and established brands that would be expected to have the *best* findings.

SURPRISING FAILURE RATES IN FOLLOWING GOOD MANUFACTURING PRACTICES

ConsumerLab.com also reported on information from the FDA (obtained by a Freedom of Information Act request) revealing that 51% of 598 US dietary supplement manufacturing facilities audited from October 1, 2018, through September 30, 2019, failed inspections and received letters of noncompliance with good manufacturing practices (GMP).[23]

The situation has been worse. The failed inspection rate in US facilities peaked at 70% in 2012. "Although an improvement over past years," says Dr Cooperman, "the most recent FDA audits show that, overall, dietary supplement manufacturers need to do a lot better." He added, "Consumers often express concern about

---

Box 1
Common problems with natural medicines sold in America

1. Tablets that won't break apart properly to release all their ingredients and therefore are much less likely to be absorbed.

2. A lack of proper labeling because they had too few or too many nutrients.

3. Deceptive labeling suggesting more ingredients than provided or components that are not even in the product at all.

4. Products containing potentially dangerous, even cancer-causing, or heavy metal contaminants.

5. A lack of voluntary warnings which could help consumers avoid potential problems, such as ingredients in amounts above known tolerable levels, and a lack of public access to adverse event reports filed by manufacturers with the FDA.

6. Faulty products left on the market due to inaction by manufacturers or "quiet" recalls announced to retailers but not to the public.

7. The illegal addition of prescription or investigational drugs, particularly those sold for "erectile dysfunction," "bodybuilding," "brain health," and "weight loss."

Table 5	
Common infractions found during FDA inspections at facilities producing natural medicines	
1. Not establishing product specifications for the identity, purity, strength, or composition of the finished dietary supplement.	25% of facilities inspected
2. Not establishing or following written procedures for quality control operations.	22%
3. Not producing batch records, which include the complete information relating to the production and control of each batch.	15%

supplement ingredients from China, but the US is doing no better than China based on this limited sampling. People may also be surprised that four out of five facilities were noncompliant in Germany, where many herbal supplements have drug status, although our own tests have also shown issues with some products from Germany."[23]

The FDA noted a median of 4 infractions at facilities that received notices, although they did not release a list of the specific violations of each facility. Nevertheless, the most common breaches have each been observed at more than 15% of noncompliant facilities (**Table 5**).[23]

ADULTERATED OR MISBRANDED PRODUCTS ARE FAR TOO COMMON

A 2015 study by the New York Attorney General concluded, "DNA testing … shows that, overall, just 21% of the test results from store brand herbal supplements verified DNA from the plants listed on the products' labels—with 79% coming up empty for DNA related to the labeled content or verifying contamination with other plant material."[24] In other words, they found that if a consumer purchased one of the tested herbal supplements, they had a four-in-five chance of being duped.

In February 2019, FDA Commissioner Dr Scott Gottlieb said, "The growth in the number of adulterated and misbranded products—including those spiked with drug ingredients not declared on their labels, misleading claims, and other risks—creates new potential dangers."[25]

CONSUMERS ARE GENERALLY UNAWARE OF THE RISKS

Science-writer Markham Heid reported, "Despite recent studies that find supplements are frequently contaminated or that the best way to get nutrients is through food, Americans' interest in supplements is only growing. And experts say many supplement users don't recognize or appreciate the risks that accompany the use of these products."[17] Dr Manson compares "the current regulatory environment to 'the Wild West.'"[17] In 2018, a study in *JAMA Network Open* reported, "From 2007 through 2016, 776 adulterated dietary supplements were identified by the FDA and 146 different dietary supplement companies were implicated."[26]

A CASE STUDY: CANNABIDIOL (CBD)

A recent example surrounds the growing popularity of cannabidiol (CBD). The market size is soaring at about 27% CAGR globally[27] with projections that "the collective market for

CBD sales in the US will surpass $20 billion [USD] by 2024."[28] The *New York Times* reports, "We are bombarded by a dizzying variety of CBD-infused products: beers, gummies, chocolates and marshmallows; lotions to rub on aching joints; oils to swallow; vaginal suppositories for 'soothing,' in one company's words, 'the area that needs it most.'"[29]

According to the *New York Times*, even CVS and Walgreens have announced plans to sell CBD products in certain states. It adds, "Many of these products are vague about what exactly CBD can do. ... Yet promises abound on the internet, where numerous articles and testimonials suggest that CBD can effectively treat not just epilepsy but also anxiety, pain, sleeplessness, Crohn's disease, arthritis, and even anger.... The FDA.... sent out a flurry of letters warning companies not to make medical claims."[29]

In 2015, an academic study reported that it found that many CBD-labeled products contained very little CBD.[30] Two years later, another study published in *JAMA* found that in 84 CBD products sold online, 36 (43%) had more CBD than advertised, and 22 (26%) had less. Also, 18 of the 84 products (21%) contained THC (the psychoactive component of marijuana), with none listed on the label, making it potentially illegal to purchase in some jurisdictions.[31]

OVERDOSING AN INCREASING ISSUE

Besides the many regulatory difficulties with natural medications, many other potential dangers exist for consumers. For example, one group of independent pharmacy professionals wrote, "Although many people don't realize it, dietary supplements can cause serious health concerns when taken incorrectly. In fact, they are a common reason for calls to U.S. Poison Control Centers, and dietary-supplement-related calls are on the rise."[32]

For example, from 2000 to 2012, US Poison Control Centers received nearly 275,000 calls related to dietary supplements (or one call every 24 minutes) with an almost 50% increase between 2005 and 2012. One in 20 calls reported a serious medical outcome, including, in rare cases, death. The majority of the calls involved miscellaneous dietary supplements, followed by botanicals and hormonal products. Of these, 70% related to dietary supplement use in children younger than 6 years old.[33] The pharmacists added, "These exposures were mostly accidental, so it's important to store dietary supplements out of the reach of children."[32]

INTERACTIONS AND TOXICITIES

Another critical issue is the possibility of the interactions and direct toxicities of natural medicines. The NCCIH warns, "Although there is a widespread public perception that herbs and botanical products in dietary supplements are safe, research has demonstrated that these products carry the same dangers as other pharmacologically active compounds. Interactions may occur between prescription drugs, over the counter drugs, dietary supplements, and even small molecules in food — making it a daunting challenge to identify all interactions that are of clinical concern."[34]

In 2019, researchers from Harvard's T.H. Chan School of Public Health found that of the single-supplement-related adverse event reports in children and young adults, "approximately 40% ... involved severe medical outcomes, including death and hospitalization; supplements sold for weight loss, muscle building, and energy were associated with almost three times the risk for severe medical outcomes compared to vitamins; and supplements sold for sexual function and colon cleanse were associated with approximately two times the risk for severe medical outcomes compared to vitamins."[35]

EVIDENCE OF EFFECTIVENESS IS USUALLY LACKING

Despite ubiquitous advertising claiming that natural medicines (as a broad category) are effective, very little reliable evidence supports most of these claims. "With a few exceptions, the research done on dietary supplements is unconvincing and largely negative."[16] The National Institute on Aging (NAI) adds, "Some advertisements for dietary supplements in magazines, online, or on TV promise that some of these products will make you feel better, keep you from getting sick, or even help you live longer. It's important to know that often, there is little, if any, science supporting these claims.[36]

HOW DID THIS COME TO BE?

Health professionals and consumers in America can rely on prescriptions and FDA-regulated over the counter medications to be high-quality, safe, and effective. The same is not true for natural medicines. Scott Gavura, writing for *Science-Based Medicine*, explains how this situation arose:[16]

"It's a consequence of legislation deliberately designed to weaken the FDA's ability to regulate and provide oversight of supplements. The Dietary Supplement Health and Education Act of 1994 (DSHEA) was an amendment to the US Federal Food, Drug, and Cosmetic Act that established the American regulatory framework for dietary supplements. It effectively *excludes* manufacturers of these products from many of the requirements that are in place for prescription and over-the-counter drugs. Amazingly, it puts the requirement to demonstrate harm on the FDA, rather than the onus on the manufacturer to show a product is safe and effective."

Natural Medicines adds:

"One of the biggest differences between drug regulations and dietary supplement regulations is the approval process. There is NO approval process for dietary supplements. As long as supplements contain dietary ingredients that were either already used in supplements before DSHEA (1994), or established as reasonably safe since then, they can be sold to consumers lawfully. This is very different from drugs, which must go through an extensive approval process BEFORE entering the market. Basically, drugs are assumed unsafe until proven safe, whereas supplements are assumed safe until proven otherwise."[37]

HEALTH PROFESSIONALS AND CONSUMERS NEED TO BE BETTER INFORMED

Unless Congress repeals or revises the DSHEA Act, the only hope for the average health professional or consumer considering recommending or using a natural medication is to ask the questions we've adapted from the PBS 2016 Frontline special, "Supplements and Safety" (**Table 6**).[38]

WHERE CAN ONE FIND TRUSTWORTHY INFORMATION? NOT THE INTERNET!

In general, the Internet is an unreliable place for people to do research on natural medicines. One *Scientific American* blog reported that among health websites, retail websites presenting information on products they were selling had the lowest level of medical accuracy (only 9%). On the other hand, government websites (.gov) and websites of national organizations (.org) had the highest level of accuracy (81 and 73%, respectively). It is problematic that even these "reputable" sources were not 100% accurate.[39]

Surprisingly, the same blog reported that educational websites (.edu sites, e-books, peer-reviewed articles) only had 50% accurate medical information. Most of the books

Table 6 Questions to ask and answer before recommending or using a natural medicine	
1. Has the product triggered any health warnings or sanctions?	• Search the FDA's website for a list of all recalls (tinyurl.com/y5kxnwbu). • ConsumerLab.com notifies its subscribers of significant warnings and recalls. • Given the few resources put into monitoring supplement safety issues, a lack of notices is no assurance of quality or safety.
2. Does the product sound too good to be true?	Supplement makers cannot legally make unfounded claims of efficacy; however, these sorts of claims regularly appear on products or the Internet. Extraordinary claims should not be believed.
3. Is there evidence that the supplement does what it promises?	Look to reputable peer-reviewed resources that summarize evidence without bias. If good evidence supporting efficacy and safety claims is not readily available, that is a giant red flag that the product may be bogus.

found by search engines either provided outdated or irrelevant information. Blogs and websites of individuals are even worse, having low rates of accuracy (26 and 30%, respectively).[39]

TRUSTWORTHY GENERAL INFORMATION

Several trustworthy, medically accurate, unbiased, and evidence-based sources of information are available at no cost and can be recommended:

1. The National Institutes of Health (NIH) has summaries about the most consumed supplements—vitamins and minerals—in a series of fact sheets.[40]
2. The US National Library of Medicine's MedlinePlus has similar information about drugs, herbs, and supplements.[41]
3. Resources are also available for specific groups. For example, the Department of Defense offers information about the safety of specific supplements for service members.[42] Older adults can find resources specifically designed for them by the FDA,[43] FTC,[44] and NIA.[36]
4. The NIH's National Center for Complementary and Integrative Health (NCCIH) provides information about complementary health products and practices—including many natural medicines.[45]

These sites can give general information on natural medicines but are of very little help when it comes to choosing specific products for specific diagnoses, especially in a highly unregulated environment.

HOW TO FIND CLINICALLY USEFUL, EVIDENCE-BASED INFORMATION?

How does a busy health professional keep up with this often-hard-to-find information about natural medicines that are safe and effective for common conditions—and affordable (another relevant factor)? The only real protection health professionals and consumers have from inaccurate information, unscrupulous manufacturers, untrained salespeople, and fraudulent, contaminated, or dangerous products is to recommend or use products that have been tested by an independent lab which makes the data available to the public.

Labs such as ConsumerLab.com, the National Sanitation Foundation (NSF International), Labdoor.com, and the United States Pharmacopeia (USP) purchase products from the marketplace (big box stores, health food stores, pharmacies, the Internet, etc.) and test them or have them tested for quality.

The two largest and oldest organizations for evidence-based information on natural medicines, including details on specific brands, are ConsumerLab.com and *Natural Medicines*. ConsumerLab.com uses a variety of labs for its tests to evaluate products, while *Natural Medicines* highlights products that are USP-Verified. Both organizations are independent of the natural medicine industrial and sales complex and make their findings and recommendations publicly available via Internet subscription. You can also get free online information from NSF, USP, and Labdoor.com about the products they have evaluated.

For over 2 decades we've recommended the constantly updated and evidence-based information from the experts in natural medicines at ConsumerLab.com and *Natural Medicines*. In our opinion, these 2 groups provide the most up-to-date, accurate information on safe, effective, and economical options to consider. Furthermore, they help people avoid potentially dangerous, unproven, and money-wasting natural medicines.[a]

ConsumerLab.com

ConsumerLab.com, LLC, founded in 1999, has been a leading provider of independent test results and information to help consumers and health professionals identify the best quality health and nutrition products. It publishes results of its tests in comprehensive reports at a subscription website, www.ConsumerLab.com, along with expert answers to many common questions about natural medicines and integrative medical practices. They frequently post news reports and information about recalls and warnings.

ConsumerLab.com claims to have "perhaps the highest testing standards of any third-party group certifying the quality of dietary supplements" and "are also the only third-party verification group that freely publishes its testing methods and quality criteria/standards." Their standard is to test products for at least 5 characteristics (**Box 2**). Products that pass all the tests are "Approved" and are eligible to bear the ConsumerLab "Seal of Approval" on their label, which "guarantees consumers the specific product carrying the Seal has met ConsumerLab's standards and passed all of ConsumerLab's tests for ingredient quality."

The ConsumerLab Seal also indicates the specific ingredients of the product that were laboratory tested by experts. In addition to the products it selects to review, ConsumerLab enables companies of all sizes to have the quality of their products tested for potential inclusion in its list of "Approved" products.

ConsumerLab gives the typical cost (in USD) of each product they review, which helps with price comparisons and helps consumers determine which products offer

---

[a] Drs Larimore and O'Mathúna indicated they do not nor ever have had any financial relationship with either publication. Dr Larimore does serve as a volunteer physician peer-reviewer for *Prescriber's Letter*.

> **Box 2**
> **ConsumerLab.com tests for the quality of a natural medication**
>
> 1. Identity: Does the product meet recognized standards of identifying all ingredients and the level of quality claimed on the label?
> 2. Strength: Does the product contain the amount of the ingredient claimed on the label?
> 3. Purity: Is the product free of specified contaminants?
> 4. Disintegration: If a tablet, does it break apart correctly so that it may be absorbed?

the best value. ConsumerLab also provides their "Top Picks" for each natural medicine tested.

Since 1999, ConsumerLab has tested more than 5600 products, representing over 850 different brands and nearly every type of popular supplements for adults, children, and pets. We consider ConsumerLab.com to be the *Consumer Reports* of natural medicines.

CASE STUDY: VITAMIN C

For example, ConsumerLab tested 31 vitamin C products in February 2020. Three failed, and 28 were "Approved." Of those "Approved," ConsumerLab chose 3 products as their "Top Picks." The cost to obtain 500 mg of vitamin C from each product they tested, based upon the price they paid, ranged from as little as 1 cent to as much as $2.80.

However, among these products, the suggested daily doses ranged from 63 mg to 5000 mg. Such a broad range provides another reason why someone should not just follow the instructions on a natural medicine label. People should choose a product that will provide the amount of vitamin C they need. ConsumerLab's "Top Picks" help do that. Their reviews also list vegan and kosher products.

NATURAL MEDICINES™

Natural Medicines, formerly known as *The Natural Medicines Comprehensive Database*, is also a subscription website and is published by independent pharmacy professionals who also publish *Prescriber's Letter*. They provide authoritative, independent, evidence-based information and resources on natural medicines as well as complementary, alternative, and integrative therapies which provide health professionals and the public with interactive tools and over 1250 monographs on the safety, effectiveness, and cautions for food, vitamins, herbs, and supplements and an additional 150 monographs on health and wellness topics. For each condition or diagnosis, *Natural Medicines* advises about each substance or therapy with 2 ratings:

1. *SAFETY*, which is broken into: "Likely Safe," "Possibly Safe," "Insufficient Evidence for Safety," "Possibly Unsafe," "Likely Unsafe," or "Unsafe." Meredith Worthington, PhD, the former Senior Editor at *Natural Medicines*, writes, "Our 'Likely Safe' rating means that an ingredient has good evidence of safe use and would generally be considered appropriate to recommend."[46]
2. *EFFECTIVENESS*: "Effective," "Likely Effective," "Possibly Effective," "Insufficient Evidence for Effectiveness," "Possibly Ineffective," "Likely Ineffective," or "Ineffective."

All ratings are based upon evidence-based, peer-reviewed, objective standards. One caution about the *Natural Medicines* ratings when it comes to their term "Possibly Effective" is, "A product might be rated 'Possibly Effective' for one condition but be rated 'Likely Ineffective' for another condition, depending on the evidence." Furthermore, by "Possibly Effective," they mean, "This product has some clinical evidence supporting its use for a specific indication; however, the evidence is limited by quantity, quality, or contradictory findings. Products rated 'Possibly Effective' might be beneficial, but do not have enough high-quality evidence to recommend for most people."[46]

Natural Medicines also has extensive information on "Health and Wellness" topics (ie, everything from "Acupressure" to "Zero Balancing"), including many complementary and alternative medicine (CAM) therapies. Their NMBER (*Natural Medicines* Brand Evidence-based Rating) rating is provided for over 185,000 commercial brand products. NMBER provides an objective, scientific rating for most commercially available natural medicines and rates each from 1 to 10, with 10 being the highest. We do not recommend any product unless it has an NMBER rating of 8 or higher. *Natural Medicines* licenses its content to WebMD. We think of *Natural Medicines* as the PDR of natural medicines.

Both organizations make most of their information available via subscription and their reviews are continually updated. Having access to one or both can provide health professionals with the latest information on these topics or products as well as other content such as the latest recalls and warnings, answers to common questions, interactions with tests or other medications, and more.

SUMMARY

In **Box 3**, we've adapted the cautions NCCIH gives health professionals and consumers when it comes to natural medications.[47]

For health professionals, having easy-to-find, objective, evidence-based, and up-to-date information on natural medicines is critical to providing quality patient care. This information must include the evidence for the safety, effectiveness, interactions, adverse effects, and appropriate condition-specific dosing for any natural medicine that is recommended to patients. At this point in time, it seems that ConsumerLab.com and *Natural Medicines* are the best sources for clinicians.

CASE STUDY: VITAMIN D

David S. Seres, MD, ScM, PNS, FASPEN.
  Dónal O'Mathúna, BSc(Pharm), MA, PhD.
  Walter L. Larimore, MD, FAAFP, DABPS.
  Vitamin D has received enormous attention in the medical literature, and supplementation has been touted for prevention of cardiovascular disease, cancer, respiratory illness, improving outcomes in the critically ill, and most recently for the prevention and treatment of COVID-19. In the aggregate, and despite the thousands of observational studies and reviews showing clear correlations, randomized trials do not support a role for vitamin D in primary or secondary prevention,[48,49] other than in the presence of deficiency. In a Cochrane systematic review and meta-analysis of randomized controlled trials (RCTs) that reported mortality, a potential for decreased mortality was seen in the elderly, likely due to a higher risk for deficiency in that population.[49] In an RCT of older adults, high dose supplementation did not prevent acute respiratory infections.[50] Moreover, there is potential for harm. In a large cohort study from the Centers for Disease Control and Prevention's (CDC) National Health and Nutrition Examination Survey (NHANES), vitamin D supplement use was associated with all-cause mortality.[51]

> **Box 3**
> **National Center for Complementary and Integrative Health (NCCIH) cautions about natural medicines**
>
> 1. The amount of scientific evidence we have on dietary supplements varies widely—we have a lot of information on some and very little on others.
> 2. Some dietary supplements can be good for your health; however, most have insufficient evidence that they are safe and effective.
> 3. Legitimate peer-reviewed studies of many supplements frequently do not support claims made about them.
> 4. Supplements you buy from stores or online often differ in important ways from products tested in studies.
> 5. Some products marketed as dietary supplements may contain prescription drugs not allowed in dietary supplements, or other ingredients or contaminants not listed on the label. Some of these ingredients may be unsafe.
> 6. The FDA does not have the resources to test all products marketed as natural medicines.
> 7. The advertising about or labels on commercially available natural medicines cannot be trusted unless certified by an independent quality testing lab.

A true deficiency occurs only when the lack of a substance causes a pathology that is reversed or prevented when the substance is replaced or supplemented. Low levels of numerous nutrients often occur because of disease activity, and do not represent deficiency. Take, for instance, the relationship between calcium and albumin. Since much of the calcium in the bloodstream is bound to albumin, a decrement in albumin causes a decrement in calcium. But this is not a deficiency, and adjustment of calcium based on albumin is taught to every medical student.

Similarly, vitamin D binding protein (VDBP), onto which most of the vitamin D in the bloodstream is bound, drops because of acute illness and systemic inflammatory response.[52] This is thought to be due to the same mechanism by which albumin drops, that is capillary leak. The sicker the patient, the greater the capillary leak and the lower the carrier protein levels. It is no surprise and indisputable, therefore, that there are strong correlations between vitamin D levels and length of stay and mortality in the critically ill,[53,54] just as there are strong associations between albumin and outcome. But only VDBP, and not free vitamin D, is correlated with ICU survival when both are measured.[55] Moreover, supplementation has failed to result in benefit in RCTs.[56,57] Thus, these reductions in vitamin D levels are disease epiphenomena, and do not represent deficiency in the critically ill.

Within the first few months of the SARS-CoV-2 pandemic, theoretic and observational studies reporting a relationship between vitamin D and COVID-19,[58] and health experts touting the potential benefits of vitamin D supplementation for the prevention and treatment of COVID-19 were making national news.[59–61] Of note, the first of these studies[58] made national news after it was made available as a preprint prior to peer review at the British Medical Journal (BMJ). It was subsequently rejected by the BMJ, and (to the best of our knowledge) has never been published in a peer reviewed journal. The growing popularity and acceptance of preprints has been a problematic development during COVID-19.[62] Evidence-based reviewers, such as the pharmacology experts at Natural Medicines, continue to say, "There is insufficient reliable evidence to rate" vitamin D for the prevention or treatment of COVID-19.[63]

Despite the clear pathophysiology for low vitamin D levels in these patients, and RCTs showing no benefit from supplementation in critical illness or COVID-19, authors continue to promote supplementation as primary prevention for these conditions and refer to low levels as "deficiency."[64]

Nevertheless, given the myriad immune mechanisms dependent on vitamin D,[65] it is highly likely that patients with true vitamin D deficiency are more likely to have worse outcomes from critical illness or COVID-19, and there may be benefit for them from supplementation.[66] But the role for population-wide supplementation with vitamin D to prevent or treat COVID-19 is far from established.

BIOGRAPHY

Dónal O'Mathúna, BSc(Pharm), MA, PhD, is Associate Professor in the College of Nursing, The Ohio State University (OSU), Columbus, Ohio, the director of the OSU Cochrane Affiliate at the Helene Fuld Health Trust National Institute for Evidence-based Practice in Nursing and Healthcare, and is on the Executive Committee, Cochrane US Network.

Walter L. Larimore, MD, FAAFP, DABPS, is a family physician, medical journalist, and best-selling author who has been listed in "The Best Doctors in America," "Distinguished Physicians of America," "Who's Who in the World," and "International Health Professionals of the Year," and who practices in Colorado Springs, Colorado.

David S. Seres, MD, ScM, PNS, FASPEN, is director of medical nutrition and associate professor of medicine in the Institute of Human Nutrition, Columbia University Medical Center, New York, NY; directs the nutrition support service, the medical school nutrition curriculum, and one of the few clinical nutrition fellowships for physicians in the US; serves as a clinical ethicist and a Columbia University/OpEd Project Public Voices Fellow; and was honored with the prestigious Excellence in Nutrition Education Award from the American Society for Nutrition.

CLINICS CARE POINTS

- Clinicians are often surprised to learn how many natural medicines (herbal remedies, dietary supplements, or vitamins) their patients are taking.
- Each patient's history should include all the natural medicines they take either regularly or as needed.
- Patients should be advised verbally and/or via handout of the potential benefits, side effects, and risks, including interactions with conditions, foods, lab tests, and/or other prescribed or over-the-counter medications they may be taking.
- If there is evidence supporting the recommendation of a natural medication for a particular patient, recommendations should also be made of specific products that have been passed or approved by an independent quality testing organization.

DISCLOSURE

None of the authors have any commercial or financial conflicts of interest. No funding source was used.

REFERENCES

1. Natural Doesn't Necessarily Mean Safer. or Better. National Center for Complementary and Integrative Health. Available at: tinyurl.com/54yv9wvb. Accessed January 31, 2022.

2. Dietary Supplements Market to Reach USD 216.3 Billion by 2026. Reports and Data. Cision PR Newswire. December 04, 2019. Available at: tinyurl.com/sduqqbo. Accessed January 31, 2022.

3. Global Dietary Supplements Market Size Will Grow USD 220.3 Billion by 2022. Zion Market Research. April 12, 2018. Available at: tinyurl.com/u9aqxor. Accessed January 31, 2022.

4. Larimore W. The natural medicines handbook: the truth about the most effective herbs, vitamins, and supplements for common conditions. Grand Rapids (MI): Revell; 2020. p. 20.

5. O'Mathúna D, Larimore W. Alternative medicine: the Christian handbook. Grand Rapids (MI): Zondervan; 2001.

6. O'Mathúna D, Larimore W. Alternative Medicine: the options, the claims, the evidence, how to choose wisely. Grand Rapids (MI): Zondervan; 2006.

7. Mole, Beth. Supplements are a $30 billion racket—here's what experts actually recommend. ARS Technica. 2018(Feb 20). Available at: tinyurl.com/yc5t22zj. Accessed January 31, 2022.

8. Natural Medicines & Supplements Database. TRC Healthcare. Available at: tinyurl.com/y2uow5cg. subscription web site, last accessed January 31, 2022.

9. CRN Reveals Initial Data from 2021 Consumer Survey on Dietary Supplements. Council for Responsible Nutrition. 2021. Available at: https://tinyurl.com/2p9c5bfe. Accessed January 31, 2022.

10. Poll finds 86% of Americans take vitamins or supplements yet only 21% have a confirmed nutritional deficiency. News Release. American Osteopathic Medical Association. 2019(Jan 16). tinyurl.com/y4g3g7lm. Accessed January 31, 2022.

11. Safdi, Alan. Vitamins and Supplements: Crucial or Superfluous? Wagner Skis Health and Wellness. Available at: tinyurl.com/y62rtqwv. Accessed January 31, 2022.

12. Dietary Supplement Use Reaches All Time High. CRN Newsroom. 2019 (Sept 30). Available at: tinyurl.com/y6y4r568. Accessed January 31, 2022.

13. Top-rated Vitamin and Supplement Brands and Merchants for 2022 Based on Consumer Satisfaction. ConsumerLab.com. 2022(Feb 25). Available at: tinyurl.com/2p82k4h2. Accessed March 14, 2022.

14. Natural Doesn't Necessarily Mean Safer, or Better. National Center for Complementary and Integrative Health. Site Last Updated January 4, 2022. Available at: tinyurl.com/rwcm9lr. Accessed January 31, 2022.

15. Hagopian J. The Evils of Big Pharma Exposed. Global Research. 2021(Sept 22). Available at: tinyurl.com/yawtm4n3. Accessed January 31, 2022.

16. Gavura S. The consumer lab rat: More questions about supplement safety. Science-Based Medicine. 2016(Jan 28). Available at: tinyurl.com/2p866ssp. Accessed January 31, 2022.

17. Heid M. The Problem with Supplements. Elemental.com. 2019(May 6). Available at: tinyurl.com/y264xawr. Accessed January 31, 2022.

18. Dietary Supplements: Sorting out the Science. Harvard Health Publishing. 2020. Available at: tinyurl.com/mr29uene. Accessed January 31, 2022.

19. Manson JE, Bassuk SS. Vitamin and Mineral Supplements: What Clinicians Need to Know. JAMA 2018;319(9):859–60. https://doi.org/10.1001/jama.2017.21012. Available at: tinyurl.com/yckhbc5u. Accessed January 31, 2022.

20. FDA clamps down on supplement claims for Alzheimer Disease. Natural Medicines. TRC Healthcare. 2019. tinyurl.com/343escny. Accessed January 31, 2022.

21. Alt DK, Anscombe AJ. Government Issues Warnings on Dietary Supplements - What's Next? Steptoe.com. 2019(Feb 20). Available at: tinyurl.com/tyrxluz. Accessed January 31, 2022.

22. Tod Cooperman. Testimony to Senate Special Committee on Aging, Subcommittee on Dietary Supplements." ConsumerLab.com. 2010(May 26). Available at: tinyurl.com/y4b4jjlb. Accessed January 31, 2022.

23. FDA Finds Problems at 52% of Supplement Manufacturing Sites in U.S. and 42% Abroad. ConsumerLab.com. 2020(Mar 13). Available at: tinyurl.com/vkhr2vu. Accessed January 31, 2022.

24. Schneiderman AG. Asks major retailers to halt sales of certain herbal supplements as DNA tests Fail to Detect plant materials listed on majority of products tested. Office of the Attorney General Press Release; 2015. Available at: tinyurl.com/wmbpkma. Accessed January 31, 2022.

25. Statement from FDA Commissioner Scott Gottlieb, M.D., on the agency's new efforts to strengthen regulation of dietary supplements by modernizing and reforming FDA's oversight. U.S. Food and Drug Administration. 2019(Feb 11). Available at: tinyurl.com/y6ss5djm. Accessed January 31, 2022.

26. Tucker J, Fischer T, Upjohn L, et al. Unapproved Pharmaceutical Ingredients Included in Dietary Supplements Associated with US Food and Drug Administration Warnings. JAMA Netw Open 2018;1(6):e183337. https://doi.org/10.1001/jamanetworkopen.2018.3337. Available at: tinyurl.com/y6dbwpp9. Accessed January 31, 2022.

27. Worldwide CBD Industry to 2025: Rising Popularity of CBD Oil is Driving Growth. Research and Markets. GlobalNewsWire.com. 2021(Dec 21). Available at: tinyurl.com/yckwxmb4. Accessed January 31, 2022.

28. Dorbian I. CBD Market Could Reach $20 Billion By 2024, Says New Study. Forbes.com. Available at: tinyurl.com/3tkhbe44, 2019. Accessed January 31, 2022.

29. Velasquez-Manoff M. Can CBD really do all that. New York Times Magazine; 2019. Available at: tinyurl.com/yymxhnax. subscription, last accessed January 31, 2022.

30. Vandrey V, Raber JC, Rabe ME, et al. Cannabinoid Dose and Label Accuracy in Edible Medical Cannabis Products. JAMA 2015;313(24):2491–3. https://doi.org/10.1001/jama.2015.6613. Available at: tinyurl.com/unsdgtb. Accessed January 31, 2022.

31. Bonn-Miller MO, Loflin MJE, Thomas BF, et al. Labeling Accuracy of Cannabidiol Extracts Sold Online. JAMA 2017;318(17):1708–9. https://doi.org/10.1001/jama.2017.11909. Available at: tinyurl.com/yb3j43uy. Accessed January 31, 2022.

32. Supplement-related calls to Poison Control Centers on the rise. Natural Medicines. TRC Healthcare. 2019(March). Available at: tinyurl.com/2sa9bktf. subscription website last accessed January 31, 2022.

33. Rao N, Spiller HA, Hodges NL, et al. An Increase in Dietary Supplement Exposures Reported to US Poison Control Centers. J Med Tox 2017;13(3):227–37. https://doi.org/10.1007/s13181-017-0623-7. Available at: tinyurl.com/wouck7h. Accessed January 31, 2022.

34. Herb-Drug Interactions. NCCIH Clinical Digest for health professionals. July 2021. Last Updated January 4, 2022. Available at: tinyurl.com/yxea8txs. Accessed January 31, 2022.

35. Or F, Kim Y, Simms J, et al. Taking Stock of Dietary Supplements' Harmful Effects on Children, Adolescents, and Young Adults. J Adol Med 2019;65(4):455–61. Available at: tinyurl.com/suo2nhz. Accessed January 31, 2022.

36. Dietary Supplements for Older Adults. NIH National Institute on Aging (NIA). Content last reviewed April 23, 2021. Available at: tinyurl.com/y53hn6hz. Accessed January 31, 2022.
37. Are dietary supplements regulated? Natural Medicines. TRC Healthcare. 2019(Jan). Available at: tinyurl.com/z72kfzaw. subscription website last accessed January 31, 2022.
38. Supplements and Safety. PBS Frontline. Episode 3. January 19, 2016. Available at: tinyurl.com/y7evl7b8. Accessed January 31, 2022.
39. Rehman J. Accuracy of Medical Information on the Internet. Guest Blog. ScientificAmerican.com. tinyurl.com/y6weu2on, 2012. Accessed January 31, 2022.
40. Vitamin and Mineral Supplement Fact Sheets. NIH Office of Dietary Supplements. Available at: tinyurl.com/nhbozqz. Accessed January 31, 2022.
41. Drugs, Herbs and Supplements. Available at: MedlinePlus.com tinyurl.com/y4euh8pn. Accessed January 31, 2022.
42. Operation Supplement Safety. Department of Defense Dietary Supplement Resource. Available at: tinyurl.com/y3fyrv39. Accessed January 31, 2022.
43. Tips for Older Dietary Supplement Users. U.S. Food and Drug Administration. Available at:tinyurl.com/y5jnept6. Accessed January 31, 2022.
44. Dietary Supplements. Consumer Information. Federal Trade Commission. Available at: tinyurl.com/yyc44hjw. Accessed January 31, 2022.
45. Worthington M. National Center for Complementary and Integrative Health (NCCIH). National Institutes for Health (NIH). Available at: tinyurl.com/uk8zjrk. Accessed January 31, 2022.
46. Worthington M. Personal email communication. July 22, 2019.
47. Using Dietary Supplements Wisely. National Center for Complementary and Integrative Health (NCCIH). National Institutes for Health (NIH). Available at: tinyurl.com/y29c2muc. Accessed January 31, 2022.
48. Manson JE, Cook NR, Lee I-M, et al. Vitamin D Supplements and Prevention of Cancer and Cardiovascular Disease. N Engl J Med 2019;380(1):33–44.
49. Bjelakovic G, Gluud LL, Nikolova D, et al. Vitamin D supplementation for prevention of cancer in adults. Cochrane Database Syst Rev 2014;(6):CD007469.
50. Camargo CA, Sluyter J, Stewart AW, et al. Effect of Monthly High-Dose Vitamin D Supplementation on Acute Respiratory Infections in Older Adults: A Randomized Controlled Trial. Clin Inf Dis 2020;71(2):311–7.
51. Chen F, Du M, Blumberg JB, et al. Association Between Dietary Supplement Use, Nutrient Intake, and Mortality Among US Adults: A Cohort Study. Ann Int Med 2019;170(9):604–13.
52. Bouillon R, Schuit F, Antonio L, et al. Vitamin D Binding Protein: A Historic Overview. Front Endocrinol (Lausanne) 2019;10:910.
53. Matthews LR, Ahmed Y, Wilson KL, et al. Worsening severity of vitamin D deficiency is associated with increased length of stay, surgical intensive care unit cost, and mortality rate in surgical intensive care unit patients. Am J Surg 2012;204(1):37–43.
54. de Haan K, Groeneveld AB, de Geus HR, et al. Vitamin D deficiency as a risk factor for infection, sepsis, and mortality in the critically ill: Systematic review and meta-analysis. Crit Care 2014;18(6):660.
55. Yoo JW, Jung YK, Ju S, et al. Serum vitamin D binding protein level, but not serum total, bioavailable, free vitamin D, is higher in 30-days survivors than in nonsurvivors with sepsis. Medicine (Baltimore) 2020;99(25):e20756.

56. Nair P, Venkatesh B, Lee P, et al. A Randomized Study of a Single Dose of Intramuscular Cholecalciferol in Critically Ill Adults. Crit Care Med 2015;43(11): 2313–20.

57. Ginde AA, Brower RG, Caterino JM, et al. Early High-Dose Vitamin D3 for Critically Ill, Vitamin D-Deficient Patients. N Engl J Med 2019;381(26):2529–40.

58. Daneshkhah A, Agrawal V, Eshein A. The Possible Role of Vitamin D in Suppressing Cytokine Storm and Associated Mortality in COVID-19 Patients. medRxiv (preprint). 2020. Available at: tinyurl.com/362ku548. Accessed January 31, 2022.

59. Frieden T. Former CDC Chief Dr. Tom Frieden: Coronavirus infection risk may be reduced by Vitamin D (opinion). Fox News. 2020(Mar 23). Available at: tinyurl.com/4uxcmdzr. Accessed January 31, 2022.

60. Sparks A. Online health gurus advise 'near-lethal' vitamin doses to combat coronavirus. New York Post. 2020(Feb 27). Available at: tinyurl.com/mr382chj. Accessed January 31, 2022.

61. Thakkar VT. Vitamin D and Coronavirus Disparities: Supplements may promote immunity, especially in people with darker skin. Wall Street Journal. 2020(Apr 16). Available at: tinyurl.com/2p8zyncx. Accessed January 31, 2022.

62. O'Mathuna DP. Ivermectin and the integrity of healthcare evidence during COVID-19. Front Pub Health. 2022;10:788972: Available at: tinyurl.com/yc8ppx3b (last Accessed March 1, 2022).

63. Vitamin D Monograph. Natural Medicines. TRC Healthcare. Last updated January 27, 2022. Available at: tinyurl.com/4abuez78. subscription website last accessed January 31, 2022.

64. Pereira M, Damascena AD, Azevedo LMG, et al. Vitamin D deficiency aggravates COVID-19: systematic review and meta-analysis. Crit Rev Food Sci Nutr 2020;(Nov 4):1–9.

65. Bilezikian JP, Bikle D, Hewison M, et al. Mechanisms in Endocrinology: Vitamin D and COVID-19. Eur J Endocrinol 2020;183(5):R133–47.

66. Amrein K, Schnedl C, Holl A, et al. Effect of high-dose vitamin D3 on hospital length of stay in critically ill patients with vitamin D deficiency: the VITdAL-ICU randomized clinical trial. JAMA 2014;312(15):1520–30.

Diet for Functional Gastrointestinal Disorders/ Disorders of Gut–Brain Interaction

Sydney Pomenti, MD, Julie Devinsky, RD,
Daniela Jodorkovsky, MD*

KEYWORDS

- Gastroesophageal reflux disease • Functional dyspepsia • Irritable bowel syndrome
- Constipation • Fiber • Dietary intervention

KEY POINTS

- Clinicians should have baseline knowledge on the health-promoting effects of nutrition and be able to provide brief and consistent information to patients with disorders of gut–brain interaction.
- A low fermentable oligosaccharide, disaccharide, monosaccharide, and polyol (FODMAP) diet should be attempted in patients with irritable bowel syndrome (IBS), preferably under the guidance of a registered dietician.
- Supplementation of soluble fiber, in particular psyllium, has been found to be efficacious in the treatment of IBS, functional constipation, and FD with minimal risk to patients.

INTRODUCTION

Dietary modulation has an obvious role in the management of gastrointestinal symptoms. The purpose of this review is to assess the high-quality data on dietary interventions to guide the management of patients with functional GI disorders. Functional GI disorders, now termed disorders of gut–brain interaction, are a heterogeneous group of disorders whose pathophysiologic mechanisms are complex and often multifactorial. Symptoms can be derived from alterations in gut neuromuscular function/motility, visceral hypersensitivity, and central nervous system dysregulation. We will review the dietary role in gastroesophageal reflux disease (GERD), functional dyspepsia (FD), irritable bowel syndrome (IBS), and functional constipation (FC).

Division of Digestive and Liver Diseases, Columbia University Irving Medical Center, 630 West 168th Street Suite 3-401, New York, NY 10032, USA
* Corresponding author.
E-mail address: Dj2470@cumc.columbia.edu

Med Clin N Am 106 (2022) 899–912
https://doi.org/10.1016/j.mcna.2022.03.005
0025-7125/22/© 2022 Elsevier Inc. All rights reserved.

GASTROESOPHAGEAL REFLUX DISEASE

GERD is defined by the presence of troublesome symptoms related to the retrograde reflux of gastric contents into the esophagus. It is one of the most common gastrointestinal disorders worldwide, with the prevalence estimated in North America at 18% to 28%.[1] The role of dietary elements in symptom generation stems from the pathophysiologic mechanisms of reflux. Certain elements in diet have been implicated in lowering the lower esophageal sphincter (LES) tone; a reduction in tone could predispose to reflux by disrupting its protective barrier function. Increased episodes of reflux during transient lower esophageal sphincter relaxations (TLESRs) may also cause GERD. Gastric distention increases TLESR frequency and duration, which may be mediated by macronutrients and portion size.[2]

The rationale behind dietary manipulation in GERD is that specific items can cause direct esophageal mucosal irritation, lower the LES tone, increase gastric distention, or elicit delay in gastric emptying.[3] **Table 1** summarizes how specific diet items may contribute to GERD symptoms. Two survey-based studies attempted to elucidate the correlation with macronutrients and GERD symptoms. Both found that participants who consumed more cholesterol, saturated fatty acids, and a higher proportion of calories from fat sources had higher GERD symptom scores.[4,5] Therefore complete elimination of all foods that could contribute to GERD is commonly recommended but without evidence. A systemic review of 16 studies that studied the effect of lifestyle intervention on GERD outcomes (using validated symptom questionnaires or esophageal pH monitoring), found insufficient evidence or conflicting results for the majority of interventions examined.[6] Accordingly, the American College of Gastroenterology (ACG) guidelines do not recommend *routine* elimination of foods that can trigger reflux.[7] However, finding a patient's individual triggers has merit. In an Italian study of 100 patients from a primary care clinic, 85% of patients self-identified at least one food trigger. After dietary elimination of their triggers, the mean GERD questionnaire scores decreased by 23%, and 45% of patients agreed to continue dietary elimination alone rather than start medication.[8] Of note, the most commonly reported triggers in this study were spicy food, chocolate, pizza, tomato, and fried foods.

Introducing dietary items that have a benefit to reduce GERD is an alternative approach. In one survey of 371 participants, a lower symptom burden was noted in those with a high fiber diet (adjusted OR 0.72, $P = .04$).[4] Addition of fiber as an intervention has been studied in two prospective studies. The first randomized 45 patients to fenugreek twice daily before a meal, H_2 blockers, or placebo for 2 weeks. Those in

Table 1 Pathophysiologic mechanisms to induce GERD	
Proposed Mechanism	**List of Dietary Targets**
Direct esophageal mucosal irritation	Acidic foods Acidic beverages Spicy foods
Reduction in LES tone	Coffee Alcohol Chocolate Mint
Increased gastric distention	Carbonated beverages Calorically dense meals Large meals
Delayed gastric emptying	Fatty meals

the fenugreek arm showed a reduction in heartburn scores on weeks 1 and 2 (16–9.5 to 7.7, $P < .001$).[9] However, those randomized to placebo also showed a reduction in symptoms on week 2 but not week 1 (20–16.7 to 13.3 $P < .01$). Psyllium husk has also been prospectively evaluated in 36 patients. Although this was not a randomized study, Morozoc and colleagues performed physiologic testing pre- and post-intervention. After initiation of psyllium 5 g three times a day for 10 days, GERD scores decreased and the number of patients who experienced heartburn went from 93% at baseline to 40% ($P < .001$). A significant reduction of reflux events was noted on reflux testing (68–42, $P < .001$).[10] Therefore, fiber supplementation may be considered to reduce GERD symptoms although larger studies are warranted.

Finally, many patients ask about other natural or dietary remedies. Some common examples include licorice root, papaya enzymes, slippery elm, and apple cider vinegar. Unfortunately, although positive anecdotal evidence exists within the collective patient narrative, there are insufficient studies, whether physiologic, symptomatic, or population based, examining their role in the pathogenesis or treatment of GERD.[11]

FUNCTIONAL DYSPEPSIA

FD is a condition defined by the presence of symptoms of postprandial fullness, early satiety, epigastric pain, or epigastric burning lasting at least 3 months.[12,13] The "functional" aspect is that these symptoms are not explained by alternative causes like peptic ulcer disease, pancreatic disease, etc. The ROME foundation further subdivides this syndrome into two subgroups, postprandial distress syndrome (PPDS) and epigastric pain syndrome (EPS).[13] Mechanistically, FD is associated with abnormalities in gastric compliance, abnormal fundus accommodation, delayed gastric emptying, and visceral hypersensitivity. Evidence is limited on dietary therapy for the treatment of FD and is not discussed by the American College of Gastroenterology and Canadian Association of Gastroenterology guidelines.[14] Nevertheless, there is some evidence that certain dietary triggers can induce FD symptoms, and thus avoidance may alleviate symptoms.

A recent systematic review identified 16 studies, mostly observational and epidemiologic, that assessed adults with FD and attempted to describe dietary associations. They found that wheat-containing foods were implicated in FD symptoms in four of the studies, but only two assessed dietary elimination, specifically of gluten.[15] Another common trigger in this review was dietary fat. However, dietary restriction of fat was not assessed as an intervention.

Prospective dietary studies in FD are sparse. Goyal et al. recently published a randomized control trial of a low fermentable oligosaccharide, disaccharide, monosaccharide, and polyol (FODMAP) diet in FD patients.[16] FODMAPs are a group of short-chain carbohydrates that are poorly absorbed in the small intestine and rapidly fermented by intestinal bacteria, exerting osmotic effects.[17] In this study, 184 patients were randomized to a low FODMAP diet versus traditional dietary advice (fat restriction and smaller frequent meals) for 4 weeks. Although both arms showed significant improvement in symptoms, there was no significant difference between the two groups (66.7% response vs 56.9%, $P = .32$). However, in a subgroup analysis of 56 patients with PPDS or bloating, low FODMAP diet (short-chain fibers) had significantly better response rates compared with traditional advice. Therefore, this group concluded that dietary therapy should be tailored according to the FD subtype and those with PPDS or bloating should be considered for a low FODMAP diet. Potter et al. attempted to elucidate which component of the FODMAP triggered FD symptoms by randomizing patients to bars containing glutan, fructan, or placebo. This was a null study due to low sample size (n = 11).[18]

Caraway oil and peppermint oil may have gastroprotective, prokinetic, and analgesic effects on the stomach.[19] Chey et al performed a randomized, placebo-controlled trial of a combination formula of caraway oil (25 mg) and L-menthol (20.75 mg) that used microsphere technology to target release in the duodenum.[20] At 24 h, the caraway/menthol arm experienced a nonsignificant 14% reduction in EPS symptoms (vs 6.9% placebo, $P = .074$) and a 9.9% reduction in PPD symptoms (vs 0.1% increase placebo, $P = .039$). However, on day 28, there were no significant differences between the drug arm and the placebo arm ($P = .23$). The authors conclude that a caraway oil/L-menthol formula can provide rapid relief in symptoms, but the long-term efficacy is less clear.

IRRITABLE BOWEL SYNDROME

IBS is defined by the Rome IV criteria as recurrent abdominal pain associated with altered bowel habits (**Fig. 1**).[13] The diagnosis should be considered in those with symptoms of abdominal pain 1 day per week for at least 3 months related to defecation, associated with a change in frequency or form of stool without red-flag symptoms.[13,21] IBS is thought to have a global prevalence of approximately 11% with even more patients undiagnosed.[22,23] IBS symptoms can often be triggered by certain foods, with more than 80% of patients associating their symptoms with eating.[24] For patients with intermittent and mild-to-moderate symptoms, diet and lifestyle modifications should be considered as first-line therapy.[25,26]

Low Fermentable Oligosaccharide, Disaccharide, Monosaccharide, and Polyol

A low FODMAP diet has been used to treat IBS patients with abdominal bloating or pain, with observational and randomized control trials showing the majority of patients experience symptomatic benefits.[24] By eliminating foods that are osmotically active and rapidly fermented by bacteria, a low FODMAP diet can decrease gas, bloating, and abdominal pain.[17,27]

Foods high in FODMAPs are common in Western diets and often eaten daily by IBS patients.[17] Fructose is a free monosaccharide in fruits, honey, and high fructose corn syrup. Fructans are oligo- and polysaccharides of fructose and occur in onions, garlic, and wheat. Polyols, including sorbitol and xylitol, are sugar alcohols found in cauliflower, mushrooms, and plums. Polyols are typically used as reduced-calorie sweeteners. Galactooligosaccharides are present in legumes, beans, Brussels sprouts, cabbage, and onions; they are rapidly fermented and induce gas formation.[17]

A low FODMAP diet eliminates all FODMAPs for 4 to 8 weeks and assesses for symptom relief.[17,28] Ideally, a full nutrition assessment should be conducted by a registered dietitian (RD) to determine whether the diet is appropriate. A provider such as an RD, with skills and dietary knowledge, is important to diet success, as evidenced by randomized control trial (RCT) data that show diet success is commonly run by RD education.[28] Moreover, RDs should monitor for nutritional adequacy while following the diet as it is lower in fiber, calcium, and B vitamins. If symptoms resolve, a systematic reintroduction, category by category, can help determine an individual's triggers.[28] For patients with little to no improvement, it should first be determined whether the patient was adherent with the diet. Other nondiet-related triggers such as stress and anxiety should also be considered.

The low FODMAP diet can pose safety concerns when done without an RD's guidance. A prolonged low FODMAP diet can adversely impact intestinal bacteria by restricting most prebiotic fiber and may have adverse effects on quality of life (ie, limited ability to eat out, costly, restrictive eating patterns).[29,30] The "FODMAP gentle"

Rome IV Criteria for Irritable Bowel Syndrome

Recurrent abdominal pain on average at least 1 day/week in the last 3 months, associated with two or more of the following criteria:

- Related to defecation
- Associated with a change in frequency of stool
- Associated with a change in form (appearance) of stool

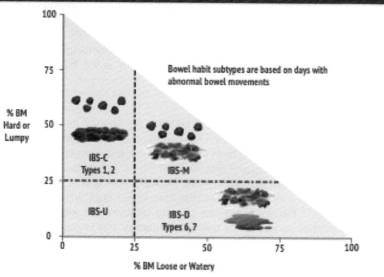

Fig. 1. Rome IV criteria for IBS, from the Rome Foundation.[13]

diet has not been as rigorously researched but is an option for patients who cannot complete the full low FODMAP diet. This includes patients with malnutrition, other dietary restrictions, comorbidities with negative risks associated with altered diet (eg, IBD and pregnancy), or poor capability to understand or apply the diet.[31] This version excludes certain foods with high FODMAP content (wheat and rye, onions, leeks, mushroom, cauliflower, milk and yogurt, apples, pears, stone fruits, dried fruits, and legumes).

Controlled studies show that gluten-free diets (GFDs) can reduce bowel frequency and decrease tight junction protein expression in the colonic mucosa of patients with diarrhea-predominant IBS (IBS-D), but there is insufficient evidence to recommend GFDs to reduce IBS symptoms.[32,33] Additionally, long-term avoidance of wheat products and can be expensive, reduce dietary fiber and iron, and also reduce *Bifidobacteria* and *Lactobacilli*.[34,35] Alterations in the gut microbiome have been hypothesized as a trigger of IBS through activation of the gut-immune system and low-grade inflammation.[36]

Lactose intolerance (LI) has a worldwide prevalence of 57% to 65%.[37] Symptoms of LI are similar to those of IBS—abdominal pain and discomfort, bloating, gas, and diarrhea. LI occurs more frequently in IBS patients, who often experience symptoms at lower lactose doses and report more severe symptoms.[38] In an RCT comparing the low FODMAP and low lactose diet, both decreased IBS severity; however, only the low FODMAP diet reduced abdominal pain and bloating.[39–42] Thus, neither the gluten free nor low lactose diets are as effective as the low FODMAP diet to treat IBS.

Soluble Fiber

The current recommendation for intake of fiber is approximately 25 to 35 g of total fiber daily, with fiber supplementation often needed to reach this recommendation.[43]

Dietary fiber is an overarching term for both soluble and insoluble fibers. Soluble fiber is made of carbohydrates and dissolves in water and includes that from psyllium, oat bran, barley, legumes, and some fruits. Insoluble fiber is from plant cell walls and does not dissolve in water; it includes that from wheat bran, whole grains, rye, and some vegetables.[44] Dietary fibers can also be differentiated into short- and long-chain carbohydrates as well as by their fermentability and viscosity. Soluble, short-chain, and fermentable dietary fibers have been found to produce gas that could aggravate symptoms of IBS, and their avoidance is discussed in the low FODMAP section. However, long-chain, soluble, viscous (gel-forming), and low fermentable dietary fibers (eg, psyllium) result in low gas production and increase stool water content.[29,45]

Soluble fibers, in particular psyllium (also referred to as Isphagula), should be considered in patients with IBS, especially those with constipation-predominant IBS. In a 2014 systematic review and meta-analysis, seven studies evaluated the use of psyllium husk in IBS.[46–52] Psyllium was found to benefit IBS symptoms with a number needed to treat of 7 (RR of IBS not improving = 0.83; 95% CI 0.73–0.94).[53] Within the same systemic review and meta-analysis, six studies evaluated insoluble, nonviscous, poorly fermentable bran with no significant benefit for IBS symptoms (overall RR of IBS not improving = 0.90; 95% CI 0.79–1.03).[52–58] Bijkerk et al randomized 275 patients with IBS (approximately half with constipation) to 10 g of psyllium versus bran versus placebo. Rates of response to treatment were higher in the psyllium group than with placebo, and symptom severity in the psyllium group was also significantly reduced compared with placebo and bran groups.[52] Early dropout was most common in the bran group, with worsening of IBS symptoms cited as main reason.

Soluble fiber supplements such as psyllium have no serious side effects and given the potential benefits should be trialed in patients with IBS.[59] Currently the ACG guidelines strongly recommend soluble but not insoluble fiber to treat IBS.[60] Psyllium supplementation should begin at a low dose (one teaspoon to one tablespoon daily) and uptitrated as some patients may experience exacerbation of symptoms including bloating and flatulence.

Prebiotics and Probiotics

Prebiotics are nondigestible foods (ie, dietary fibers) that are selectively digested by particular microorganisms and are supplemented to alter the overall gut microbiota. These include soluble, nonviscous, fermentable fibers such as inulin, fructooligosaccharides, and galactooligosaccharides[61] Prebiotics including inulin made from chicory root have been evaluated in smaller pilot studies. Some studies showed improvement in IBS symptoms; however, responses have been mixed and dose dependent even in small studies.[62–64] Larger RCTs are needed.

Probiotics are live microorganisms, which are supplemented for potential health benefits, including the possibility that they may improve the balance of the gut microbiota.[65] Strains of lactic acid bacilli including Bifidobacterium and Lactobacillus are some of the most frequently used organisms in commercial products.[65] A variety of probiotics have been studied in smaller single-center studies with poor evidence to suggest benefits. Systematic reviews and meta-analyses have not shown evidence for probiotic efficacy in IBS.[66–68] The ACG conditionally suggests against probiotics for the treatment of IBS symptoms.[60]

Peppermint

As discussed previously, patients often seek natural remedies as treatments, and peppermint oil is one of the most popular for IBS. There have been several RCTs published on a variety of formulations of peppermint oil. In the meta-analysis by Alammar and colleagues, twelve RCTs involving 835 patients were included showing that peppermint oil is a safe and effective therapy for abdominal pain and global symptoms in patients with IBS. The studies overall showed a number needed to treat of three for global symptoms and four for abdominal pain.[69] Although there are few adverse results, L-menthol that is a main component of peppermint oil may exacerbate heartburn, and therefore many trials have used enteric-coated formulations for delayed release in the small intestine.[70–74] Given the minimal risks and overall positive results in the RCTs, the ACG conditionally suggests the use of peppermint oil, with emphasis to be placed for further trials focusing on optimal formulation and benefits for the different IBS subgroups.[60]

FUNCTIONAL CONSTIPATION

FC is defined by the Rome IV as having two or more of the following for at least 25% of defecations: straining, Bristol Stool Scale 1 to 2 bowel movements (**Fig. 2**), incomplete evacuation, anorectal obstruction/blockage, manual maneuvers to facilitate defecation as well as fewer than three bowel movements per week. Additionally, loose stools are rarely present without laxative use, and there must be insufficient criteria for IBS.[13] These symptoms must be present for at least 3 months. FC has a prevalence of approximately 14%, with even high rates in women and older individuals.[75]

Fiber is considered a first-line recommendation for FC. In one metanalysis, three RCTs using various soluble fibers found soluble fiber to be beneficial compared with placebo with a number needed to treat of 2 (95% CI 1.6–3).[76] Additionally, several RCTs using psyllium were found to be effective at improving constipation.[77–79] In a recently published review, psyllium was found to be 3.4 times more effective at increasing stool output than wheat bran. Additionally, both psyllium and coarse wheat bran increased stool water content; however, ground wheat bran decreased stool water contents paradoxically causing harder stools.[80] All fibers, but in particular soluble fiber, is effective in the management of FC and should be titrated up slowly with doses limited by flatulence, bloating, and cramping that are typically worse with insoluble fiber.

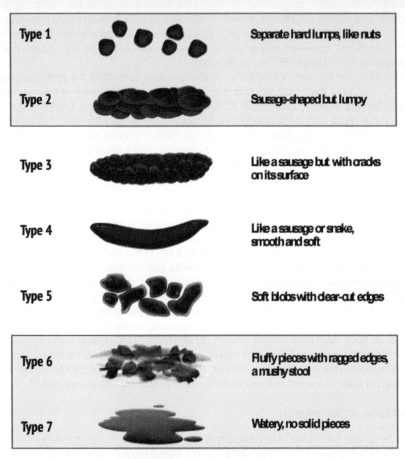

Fig. 2. Bristol stool form scale, from the Rome Foundation.[13]

Fruit-Based Laxatives for Chronic Constipation

In addition to fiber supplements, fruit-based laxatives with soluble and insoluble fibers and sugars have also been studied for chronic constipation, including both FC and IBS-C. In a randomized, double-blind, placebo-controlled trial of 87 people with FC, Kivia powder, an extract of kiwifruit, was significantly more effective than placebo at increasing spontaneous bowel movement frequency and reducing flatulence, urgency, and abdominal pain.[81] An additional randomized controlled study focusing on two kiwifruits per day in patients with IBS-C found improvements in colon transit time using Sitzmarkers and increased defecation frequency in the group consuming kiwifruit. An additional small study (n = 11) found intake of kiwifruits associated with more bowel movements with looser stools without additional bloating or changes in intestinal gas transit and tolerance.[82]

In an RCT comparing prunes to psyllium for FC, prunes significantly increased the number of spontaneous bowel movements per week and stool consistency scores compared with psyllium. Significant improvements in straining were seen in both prunes and psyllium from baseline, and both were considered palatable.[83] In a pilot study of 36 patients with chronic constipation, mango significantly improved stool frequency, consistency, and shape.[84] Chey and colleagues, recently published an RCT in which 79 patients with FC or IBS-C, were randomized to two Kiwifruits per day, 100 g of prunes grams/d, or 12 g/d of psyllium for 4 weeks. In all three treatments, there was a significant increase in complete spontaneous bowel movements and improvements in straining. Stool consistency significantly improved with kiwifruit and prunes, and patients randomized to the kiwifruit group reported significant improvement in bloating scores and the lowest rates of adverse events and dissatisfaction with treatment.[85]

CLINICS CARE POINTS

- For patients with GERD, identification and elimination of patient's individual triggers are a preferred strategy over elimination of all foods that can trigger reflux.
- In patients with FD and IBS, caraway oil and peppermint oil can be trialed for symptoms as well as a low FODMAP diet.
- Patients with IBS-D should be assessed for LI and celiac disease. If neither condition is present, neither GFD nor low lactose diet is as effective as a low FODMAP diet to treat IBS.
- Initiating patients on a low FODMAP diet should be for 4 to 8 weeks to assess symptom relief, with the goal of reintroduction of foods under the supervision of an RD.
- In patients with IBS-C and FC, supplementation of psyllium or fruit-based laxatives, including prunes and kiwifruit, should be considered.

DISCLOSURE

None of the authors have any commercial or financial conflicts of interest. No funding source was used.

REFERENCES

1. El-Serag HB, Sweet S, Winchester CC, et al. Update on the epidemiology of gastro-oesophageal reflux disease: a systematic review. Gut 2014;63(6):871–80.
2. Kim HI, Hong SJ, Han JP, et al. Specific movement of esophagus during transient lower esophageal sphincter relaxation in gastroesophageal reflux disease. J Neurogastroenterol Motil 2013;19(3):332–7.
3. Newberry C, Lynch K. The role of diet in the development and management of gastroesophageal reflux disease: why we feel the burn. J Thorac Dis 2019; 11(Suppl 12):S1594–601.

4. El-Serag HB, Satia JA, Rabeneck L. Dietary intake and the risk of gastro-oesophageal reflux disease: a cross sectional study in volunteers. Gut 2005; 54(1):11–7.

5. Shapiro M, Green C, Bautista JM, et al. Assessment of dietary nutrients that influence perception of intra-oesophageal acid reflux events in patients with gastro-oesophageal reflux disease. Aliment Pharmacol Ther 2007;25(1):93–101.

6. Kaltenbach T, Crockett S, Gerson LB. Are lifestyle measures effective in patients with gastroesophageal reflux disease? An evidence-based approach. Arch Intern Med 2006;166(9):965–71.

7. Vaezi MF, Pandolfino JE, Vela MF. ACG clinical guideline: diagnosis and management of achalasia. Am J Gastroenterol 2013;108(8):1238–49 [quiz: 1250].

8. Tosetti C, Savarino E, Benedetto E, et al. Study Group for the Evaluation of GERD Triggering Foods. Elimination of dietary triggers is successful in treating symptoms of gastroesophageal reflux disease. Dig Dis Sci 2021;66(5):1565–71.

9. DiSilvestro RA, Verbruggen MA, Offutt EJ. Anti-heartburn effects of a fenugreek fiber product. Phytother Res 2011;25(1):88–91.

10. Morozov S, Isakov V, Konovalova M. Fiber-enriched diet helps to control symptoms and improves esophageal motility in patients with non-erosive gastroesophageal reflux disease. World J Gastroenterol 2018;24(21):2291–9.

11. Ahuja A, Ahuja NK. Popular remedies for esophageal symptoms: a critical appraisal. Curr Gastroenterol Rep 2019;21(8):39.

12. Stanghellini V, Chan FKL, Hasler WL, et al. Gastroduodenal disorders. Gastroenterology 2016;150(6):1380–92.

13. Rome IV Criteria - Rome Foundation. Available at: https://theromefoundation.org/rome-iv/rome-iv-criteria/. Accessed April 18, 2021.

14. Moayyedi P, Lacy BE, Andrews CN, et al. ACG and CAG clinical guideline: management of dyspepsia. Am J Gastroenterol 2017;112(7):988–1013.

15. Duncanson KR, Talley NJ, Walker MM, et al. Food and functional dyspepsia: a systematic review. J Hum Nutr Diet 2018;31(3):390–407.

16. Goyal O, Nohria S, Batta S, et al. Low fermentable oligosaccharides, disaccharides, monosaccharides, and polyols diet versus traditional dietary advice for functional dyspepsia: a randomized controlled trial. J Gastroenterol Hepatol 2021. https://doi.org/10.1111/jgh.15694.

17. Shepherd SJ, Lomer MCE, Gibson PR. Short-chain carbohydrates and functional gastrointestinal disorders. Am J Gastroenterol 2013;108(5):707–17.

18. Potter MDE, Duncanson K, Jones MP, et al. Wheat sensitivity and functional dyspepsia: a pilot, double-blind, randomized, placebo-controlled dietary crossover trial with novel challenge protocol. Nutrients 2020;12(7).

19. May B, Köhler S, Schneider B. Efficacy and tolerability of a fixed combination of peppermint oil and caraway oil in patients suffering from functional dyspepsia. Aliment Pharmacol Ther 2000;14(12):1671–7.

20. Chey WD, Lacy BE, Cash BD, et al. A novel, duodenal-release formulation of a combination of caraway oil and l-menthol for the treatment of functional dyspepsia: a randomized controlled trial. Clin Transl Gastroenterol 2019;10(4): e00021.

21. Mearin F, Lacy BE, Chang L, et al. Bowel Disorders. Gastroenterology 2016. https://doi.org/10.1053/j.gastro.2016.02.031.

22. Lovell RM, Ford AC. Global prevalence of and risk factors for irritable bowel syndrome: a meta-analysis. Clin Gastroenterol Hepatol 2012;10(7):712–21.e4.

23. Hungin APS, Chang L, Locke GR, et al. Irritable bowel syndrome in the United States: prevalence, symptom patterns and impact. Aliment Pharmacol Ther 2005;21(11):1365–75.
24. Liu J, Chey WD, Haller E, et al. Low-FODMAP diet for irritable bowel syndrome: what we know and what we have yet to learn. Annu Rev Med 2020;71:303–14.
25. Böhn L, Störsrud S, Liljebo T, et al. Diet low in FODMAPs reduces symptoms of irritable bowel syndrome as well as traditional dietary advice: a randomized controlled trial. Gastroenterology 2015;149(6):1399–407.e2.
26. Hookway C, Buckner S, Crosland P, et al. Irritable bowel syndrome in adults in primary care: summary of updated NICE guidance. BMJ 2015;350:h701.
27. Gibson PR, Shepherd SJ. Evidence-based dietary management of functional gastrointestinal symptoms: The FODMAP approach. J Gastroenterol Hepatol 2010;25(2):252–8.
28. McKenzie YA, Bowyer RK, Leach H, et al. British Dietetic Association systematic review and evidence-based practice guidelines for the dietary management of irritable bowel syndrome in adults (2016 update). J Hum Nutr Diet 2016;29(5): 549–75.
29. Eswaran S, Muir J, Chey WD. Fiber and functional gastrointestinal disorders. Am J Gastroenterol 2013;108(5):718–27.
30. Staudacher HM. Nutritional, microbiological and psychosocial implications of the low FODMAP diet. J Gastroenterol Hepatol 2017;32(Suppl 1):16–9.
31. Halmos EP, Gibson PR. Controversies and reality of the FODMAP diet for patients with irritable bowel syndrome. J Gastroenterol Hepatol 2019;34(7):1134–42.
32. Dionne J, Ford AC, Yuan Y, et al. A systematic review and meta-analysis evaluating the efficacy of a gluten-free diet and a low FODMAPs diet in treating symptoms of irritable bowel syndrome. Am J Gastroenterol 2018;113(9):1290–300.
33. Vazquez-Roque MI, Camilleri M, Smyrk T, et al. A controlled trial of gluten-free diet in patients with irritable bowel syndrome-diarrhea: effects on bowel frequency and intestinal function. Gastroenterology 2013;144(5):903–11.e3.
34. Bellini M, Tonarelli S, Nagy AG, et al. Low FODMAP diet: evidence, doubts, and hopes. Nutrients 2020;12(1). https://doi.org/10.3390/nu12010148.
35. Shepherd SJ, Gibson PR. Nutritional inadequacies of the gluten-free diet in both recently-diagnosed and long-term patients with coeliac disease. J Hum Nutr Diet 2013;26(4):349–58.
36. Ohman L, Simrén M. Pathogenesis of IBS: role of inflammation, immunity and neuroimmune interactions. Nat Rev Gastroenterol Hepatol 2010;7(3):163–73.
37. Catanzaro R, Sciuto M, Marotta F. Lactose intolerance: An update on its pathogenesis, diagnosis, and treatment. Nutr Res 2021;89:23–34.
38. Varjú P, Farkas N, Hegyi P, et al. Low fermentable oligosaccharides, disaccharides, monosaccharides and polyols (FODMAP) diet improves symptoms in adults suffering from irritable bowel syndrome (IBS) compared to standard IBS diet: A meta-analysis of clinical studies. PLoS One 2017;12(8):e0182942.
39. Krieger-Grübel C, Hutter S, Hiestand M, et al. Treatment efficacy of a low FODMAP diet compared to a low lactose diet in IBS patients: A randomized, crossover designed study. Clin Nutr ESPEN 2020;40:83–9.
40. Reynolds A, Mann J, Cummings J, et al. Carbohydrate quality and human health: a series of systematic reviews and meta-analyses. Lancet 2019;393(10170): 434–45.
41. Johnson CM, Wei C, Ensor JE, et al. Meta-analyses of colorectal cancer risk factors. Cancer Causes Control 2013;24(6):1207–22.

42. Peters U, Sinha R, Chatterjee N, et al. Dietary fibre and colorectal adenoma in a colorectal cancer early detection programme. Lancet 2003;361(9368):1491–5.
43. U.S. Department of Health and Human Services and U.S. Department of Agriculture. 2015-2020. Dietary Guidelines for Americans. 2015. Available at: https://health.gov/our-work/food-nutrition/previous-dietary-guidelines/2015. Accessed November 27, 2021.
44. Food and Drug Administration. Food Labeling: Revision of the Nutrition and Supplement Facts Labels. Federal Register. 2016. Available at: https://www.federalregister.gov/documents/2016/05/27/2016-11867/food-labeling-revision-of-the-nutrition-and-supplement-facts-labels. Accessed November 28, 2021.
45. Chutkan R, Fahey G, Wright WL, et al. Viscous versus nonviscous soluble fiber supplements: mechanisms and evidence for fiber-specific health benefits. J Am Acad Nurse Pract 2012;24(8):476–87.
46. Ritchie JA, Truelove SC. Treatment of irritable bowel syndrome with lorazepam, hyoscine butylbromide, and ispaghula husk. Br Med J 1979;1(6160):376–8.
47. Longstreth GF, Fox DD, Youkeles L, et al. Psyllium therapy in the irritable bowel syndrome. A double-blind trial. Ann Intern Med 1981;95(1):53–6.
48. Arthurs Y, Fielding JF. Double blind trial of ispaghula/poloxamer in the Irritable Bowel Syndrome. Ir Med J 1983;76(5):253.
49. Nigam P, Kapoor KK, Rastog CK, et al. Different therapeutic regimens in irritable bowel syndrome. J Assoc Physicians India 1984;32(12):1041–4.
50. Prior A, Whorwell PJ. Double blind study of ispaghula in irritable bowel syndrome. Gut 1987;28(11):1510–3.
51. Jalihal A, Kurian G. Ispaghula therapy in irritable bowel syndrome: improvement in overall well-being is related to reduction in bowel dissatisfaction. J Gastroenterol Hepatol 1990;5(5):507–13.
52. Bijkerk CJ, de Wit NJ, Muris JWM, et al. Soluble or insoluble fibre in irritable bowel syndrome in primary care? Randomised placebo controlled trial. BMJ 2009;339:b3154.
53. Moayyedi P, Quigley EMM, Lacy BE, et al. The effect of fiber supplementation on irritable bowel syndrome: a systematic review and meta-analysis. Am J Gastroenterol 2014;109(9):1367–74.
54. Soltoft J, Krag B, Gudmand-Hoyer E, et al. A double-blind trial of the effect of wheat bran on symptoms of irritable bowel syndrome. Lancet 1976;1(7954):270–2.
55. Manning AP, Heaton KW, Harvey RF. Wheat fibre and irritable bowel syndrome. A controlled trial. Lancet 1977;2(8035):417–8.
56. Kruis W, Weinzierl M, Schüssler P, et al. Comparison of the therapeutic effect of wheat bran, mebeverine and placebo in patients with the irritable bowel syndrome. Digestion 1986;34(3):196–201.
57. Lucey MR, Clark ML, Lowndes J, et al. Is bran efficacious in irritable bowel syndrome? A double blind placebo controlled crossover study. Gut 1987;28(2):221–5.
58. Rees G, Davies J, Thompson R, et al. Randomised-controlled trial of a fibre supplement on the symptoms of irritable bowel syndrome. J R Soc Promot Health 2005;125(1):30–4.
59. Rao SSC, Yu S, Fedewa A. Systematic review: dietary fibre and FODMAP-restricted diet in the management of constipation and irritable bowel syndrome. Aliment Pharmacol Ther 2015;41(12):1256–70.
60. Lacy BE, Pimentel M, Brenner DM, et al. ACG clinical guideline: management of irritable bowel syndrome. Am J Gastroenterol 2021;116(1):17–44.

61. Gibson GR, Hutkins R, Sanders ME, et al. Expert consensus document: The International Scientific Association for Probiotics and Prebiotics (ISAPP) consensus statement on the definition and scope of prebiotics. Nat Rev Gastroenterol Hepatol 2017;14(8):491–502.

62. Silk DBA, Davis A, Vulevic J, et al. Clinical trial: the effects of a trans-galactooligosaccharide prebiotic on faecal microbiota and symptoms in irritable bowel syndrome. Aliment Pharmacol Ther 2009;29(5):508–18.

63. Isakov V, Pilipenko V, Shakhovskaya A, et al. Efficacy of inulin enriched yogurt on bowel habits in patients with irritable bowel syndrome with constipation: a pilot study. FASEB J 2013;27(S1). https://doi.org/10.1096/fasebj.27.1_supplement. lb426.

64. Wilson B, Whelan K. Prebiotic inulin-type fructans and galacto-oligosaccharides: definition, specificity, function, and application in gastrointestinal disorders. J Gastroenterol Hepatol 2017;32(Suppl 1):64–8.

65. Isolauri E, Salminen S, Ouwehand AC. Microbial-gut interactions in health and disease. Probiotics Best Pract Res Clin Gastroenterol 2004;18(2):299–313.

66. Parker EA, Roy T, D'Adamo CR, et al. Probiotics and gastrointestinal conditions: An overview of evidence from the Cochrane Collaboration. Nutrition 2018;45: 125–34.e11.

67. Brenner DM, Moeller MJ, Chey WD, et al. The utility of probiotics in the treatment of irritable bowel syndrome: a systematic review. Am J Gastroenterol 2009; 104(4):1033–49 [quiz: 1050].

68. Ford AC, Harris LA, Lacy BE, et al. Systematic review with meta-analysis: the efficacy of prebiotics, probiotics, synbiotics and antibiotics in irritable bowel syndrome. Aliment Pharmacol Ther 2018;48(10):1044–60.

69. Alammar N, Wang L, Saberi B, et al. The impact of peppermint oil on the irritable bowel syndrome: a meta-analysis of the pooled clinical data. BMC Complement Altern Med 2019;19(1):21.

70. Merat S, Khalili S, Mostajabi P, et al. The effect of enteric-coated, delayed-release peppermint oil on irritable bowel syndrome. Dig Dis Sci 2010;55(5):1385–90.

71. Ford AC, Talley NJ, Spiegel BMR, et al. Effect of fibre, antispasmodics, and peppermint oil in the treatment of irritable bowel syndrome: systematic review and meta-analysis. BMJ 2008;337:a2313.

72. Cappello G, Spezzaferro M, Grossi L, et al. Peppermint oil (Mintoil) in the treatment of irritable bowel syndrome: a prospective double blind placebo-controlled randomized trial. Dig Liver Dis 2007;39(6):530–6.

73. Liu JH, Chen GH, Yeh HZ, et al. Enteric-coated peppermint-oil capsules in the treatment of irritable bowel syndrome: a prospective, randomized trial. J Gastroenterol 1997;32(6):765–8.

74. Cash BD, Epstein MS, Shah SM. A novel delivery system of peppermint oil is an effective therapy for irritable bowel syndrome symptoms. Dig Dis Sci 2016;61(2): 560–71.

75. Suares NC, Ford AC. Prevalence of, and risk factors for, chronic idiopathic constipation in the community: systematic review and meta-analysis. Am J Gastroenterol 2011;106(9):1582–91 [quiz: 1581, 1592].

76. Ford AC, Moayyedi P, Lacy BE, et al. American College of Gastroenterology monograph on the management of irritable bowel syndrome and chronic idiopathic constipation. Am J Gastroenterol 2014;109(Suppl 1):S2–26 [quiz: S27].

77. Fenn GC, Wilkinson PD, Lee CE, et al. A general practice study of the efficacy of Regulan in functional constipation. Br J Clin Pract 1986;40(5):192–7.

78. Odes HS, Madar Z. A double-blind trial of a celandin, aloevera and psyllium laxative preparation in adult patients with constipation. Digestion 1991;49(2):65–71.
79. Ashraf W, Park F, Lof J, et al. Effects of psyllium therapy on stool characteristics, colon transit and anorectal function in chronic idiopathic constipation. Aliment Pharmacol Ther 1995;9(6):639–47.
80. McRorie JW, Fahey GC, Gibb RD, et al. Laxative effects of wheat bran and psyllium: Resolving enduring misconceptions about fiber in treatment guidelines for chronic idiopathic constipation. J Am Assoc Nurse Pract 2020;32(1):15–23.
81. Udani JK, Bloom DW. Effects of Kivia powder on gut health in patients with occasional constipation: a randomized, double-blind, placebo-controlled study. Nutr J 2013;12:78.
82. Caballero N, Benslaiman B, Ansell J, et al. The effect of green kiwifruit on gas transit and tolerance in healthy humans. Neurogastroenterol Motil 2020;32(9): e13874.
83. Attaluri A, Donahoe R, Valestin J, et al. Randomised clinical trial: dried plums (prunes) vs. psyllium for constipation. Aliment Pharmacol Ther 2011;33(7):822–8.
84. Venancio VP, Kim H, Sirven MA, et al. Polyphenol-rich Mango (Mangifera indica L.) Ameliorate Functional Constipation Symptoms in Humans beyond Equivalent Amount of Fiber. Mol Nutr Food Res 2018;62(12):e1701034.
85. Chey SW, Chey WD, Jackson K, et al. Exploratory comparative effectiveness trial of green kiwifruit, psyllium, or prunes in US patients with chronic constipation. Am J Gastroenterol 2021;116(6):1304–12.

Nutrition Resources for Patients and Providers

Melissa Townsend, MS, RD, CDN[a], Nicole Kuerzi, BS, RD, CDN, CNSC[a],
Gina DiFusco, BS, RD, CDN[a], Michelle Christensen, MS, RD, CDN, CNSC[b],
Elizabeth Miracle, MS, RD, CSO, CDN, CNSC[a,*]

KEYWORDS

- Nutrition • Nutrition education • Medical nutrition therapy • Patient education
- Registered Dietitian

KEY POINTS

- Registered Dietitians are an important patient and provider resource to furnish evidence-based nutrition care to patients, families, and caregivers.
- Preparing for patient encounters by understanding and determining a patient's language, regional dialect, cultural background, and religious preference can help guide your nutrition education and positively affect care.
- There are a variety of both patient and provider nutrition education resources available and selecting the best, most appropriate resource is vital to effective education.
- Disease-specific nutrition education materials developed by credible organizations are available to health care providers for use with patients and can serve as a way to tailor care to address individual patient needs.
- Patients requiring nutrition support should be referred to an infusion company or a durable medical equipment provider that adheres to published safe practices and is capable of meeting the needs of complex patients. Insurance coverage varies from payer to payer, and it is important to know coverage and costs when selecting an appropriate nutrition intervention.

INTRODUCTION

Patient access to appropriate, disease-specific, individualized nutrition information is imperative to help manage health outcomes and disease. As a provider, engaging in a meaningful discussion regarding nutrition and sharing appropriate resources can foster patient empowerment regarding their health; this is especially important in the age

---

Financial Disclosures: None.
[a] Department of Food and Nutrition, NewYork Presbyterian-Columbia University Irving Medical Center, 177 Fort Washington Avenue, New York, NY 10032, USA; [b] Coram® CVS Specialty® Infusion Services (Coram) 48-23 55th Avenue, Queens, NY 11378, USA
* Corresponding author. Department of Food and Nutrition, NewYork Presbyterian-Columbia University Irving Medical Center, 177 Fort Washington Avenue, New York, NY 10032.
E-mail address: eam9018@nyp.org

Med Clin N Am 106 (2022) 913–927
https://doi.org/10.1016/j.mcna.2022.03.006
0025-7125/22/© 2022 Elsevier Inc. All rights reserved.

medical.theclinics.com

of technology and connectedness, where there is a need to dispel health misinformation. In addition, this engagement can serve as a positive complement to the preventive or reactive health services that are already being provided.

When directly providing nutrition education resources or when referring patients to a qualified nutrition professional who provides medical nutrition therapy, it is efficacious to consider that there is no one-size-fits-all approach to health. The purpose of this article is to discuss the value that qualified nutrition professionals add as a complement to patient care, as well as to provide tangible resources that can be used by any health care practitioner who is tailoring nutrition education to meet an individual patient's specific needs.

WHAT IS A REGISTERED DIETITIAN?

Registered Dietitians (RDs) are widely recognized to be nutrition experts.[1] They serve as an integral component to preventive and disease-specific care in the health care setting, as well as in sports, private practice, research, community, public health, and food and nutrition–related business or industries.[1] RDs work with patients, families, and caregivers to provide personalized recommendations that connect the individual's unique medical history, medications, and laboratory values to improve diet quality, overall health, and most importantly, to meet the patient's goals. RDs are unique compared with other nutrition professionals based on the training they undergo as well as the comprehensive medical nutrition therapy (MNT) services they provide.[2] Although all RDs are nutritionists, not all nutritionists are RDs.[3,4] The rigorous training that RDs complete enables them to provide individualized, evidence-based nutrition care.

In order to attain the RD credential, individuals must undergo comprehensive academic training through undergraduate and/or graduate degree coursework in an Accreditation Council for Education in Nutrition and Dietetics (ACEND) program. After successful completion of didactic coursework, prospective dietetics practitioners are then eligible to apply for an ACEND-accredited Dietetic Internship (DI) program.[1,4,5] Once accepted to a DI, prospective dietetic practitioners complete a minimum of 1200 hours of supervised practice, to develop and hone professional skills. After completing a DI program, eligible professionals are then able to sit for a national professional examination through the Commission of Dietetics Registration (CDR), the credentialing agency for the Academy of Nutrition and Dietetics (AND).[6] Credentialing nutrition and dietetics practitioners through CDR serves to demonstrate the competency of dietetics practitioners while also protecting the public from health misinformation.[6] In addition to registration through CDR, 48 states, as well as Puerto Rico and the District of Columbia, have additional certification and licensing requirements to establish professional competence in the area of nutrition.[7]

Similar to other allied health professionals, RDs must complete 75 hours of continuing education credits over a 5-year period to continue to build on their foundational knowledge and remain up to date on new research. RDs also adhere to Standards of Practice in Nutrition Care[8,9] and Professional Performance, as well as a Code of Ethics.[10]

Services Registered Dietitians Provide

As previously discussed, RDs provide safe, evidence-based MNT to patients, families, and designated caregivers. Medical Nutrition Therapy services provided by an RD differ from just provision of nutrition education. The Academy of Nutrition and Dietetics defines nutrition education as "reinforcement of basic or essential nutrition-related knowledge."[2] MNT services include the Nutrition Care Process, which entails the Dietitian performing in-depth individualized nutrition assessment, nutrition diagnosis, intervention, and monitoring/evaluation criteria for clinical or behavioral outcomes.[2,11] MNT is evidence based, and RDs work to support lifestyle changes and address behavioral management skills to meet the patient's specific goals; this includes nutrition counseling techniques as well as implementation of theories of behavior change, including such techniques as motivational interviewing, to personalize care. Other nutrition professionals, depending on state licensure, may only be able to provide nonmedical nutrition information. Reimbursement for MNT services furnished by RDs varies from state to state and is beyond the scope of this article.

Specialized Nutrition Providers

Similar to other health care professionals, RDs are able to specialize through exposure to specific patient populations and demonstrated competency through completion of board examinations. Providers should feel confident that when they are referring patients for MNT to an RD, with or without advanced certifications, the patient will receive evidence-based, safe, and personalized care using the nutrition care process to improve health and disease outcomes. An overview of credentials that a qualified provider may possess is outlined in **Table 1**.

Finding a Qualified Nutrition Provider

RDs and those with specialized credentials to refer patients to can be found using the AND website[21] as shown in **Table 2**. RDs are also frequently affiliated with health care institutions; check with your local health care network to see if there is an RD providing ambulatory nutrition services whom you can refer your patient to. Respective insurance providers can also be used to find in-network providers.

Important things to consider when selecting a nutrition provider for referral:

- What educational background and credentials does he/she/they hold that make them qualified to provide services to my patient?
- What is his/hers/their experience level with providing nutrition care/MNT specific to my patient's disease state?
- Does he/she/they have the capability to provide nutrition care/MNT in the patient's preferred language?
- In what format is he/she/they providing nutrition care/MNT (in person vs remote)?

SELECTING APPROPRIATE EDUCATION MATERIALS

When providing nutrition education to patients, it is imperative that providers understand the individual needs of the specific patient. Although RDs, as previously discussed, receive extensive education that includes how to implement theories of behavior change and how to use motivational interviewing to personalize education, there are numerous first steps that need to be considered by any practitioner providing nutrition education.

General Recommendations

Before providing physical resources, it is important to understand what the patient's baseline knowledge is on the topic being discussed. Asking questions to learn more about what the patient's perceptions are regarding the information can be helpful in determining what level of detail they are ready to learn and accept. As a component of this, it is important to understand where patients are currently getting nutrition information from. Examples of questions to ask are as follows:

Table 1
Overview of Advanced Certifications Held by Registered Dietitians

Advanced Credential	Cedentialing Provider	Area of Expertise
Advanced Practioner Certification in Clinical Nutrition® (AP-RD)®[12]	CDR	Clinical Nutrition Care
Certified Lactation Counselor® (CLC®)[13]	ALPP	Lactation
Certified Diabetes Care Education Specialist (CDCES)[14]	CBDCE	Diabetes
Certified Eating Disorder Registered Dietitian (CEDRD)[15]	iaedp™	Eating Disorders
Certified Specialist in Gerontological Nutrition™ (CSG™)[16,17]	CDR	Gerontological Nutrition
International Board Certified Lactation Consultant® (IBCLC®)[18]	IBLCE	Lactation
Certified Nutrition Support Clinician® (CNSC®)[19]	NBNSC	Nutrition Support(Enteral/Parental nutrition)
Certified Specialist in Obesity and Weight Management™ (CSOWM™)[16,17]	CDR	Obesity and Weight Management
Certified Specialist in Oncology Nutrition™ (CSO™)[16,17]	CDR	Oncology Nutrition
Certified Specialist in Pediatric Nutrition™ (CSP™)[16,17]	CDR	Pediatric Nutrition
Certified Specialist in Pediatric Critical Care (CSP-CC™)[16,17]	CDR	Pediatric Critical Care
Certified Specialist in Renal Nutrition (CSR™)[16,17]	CDR	Renal Disease/Nephrology
Certified Specialist in Sports Dietetics™ (CSSD™)[16,17]	CDR	Sports Nutrition
Certified Clinical Transplant Dietitian (CCTD)[20]	NATCO	Transplant Nutrition

Abbreviations: ALPP, Academy of Lactation Policy and Practice; CBDCE, Certification Board for Diabetes Care and Education; CDR, Commission on Dietetics Registration; IAEDP, International Association of Eating Disorders Professionals; IBLCE, International Board of Lactation Consultant Examiners; NATCO, North American Transplant Coordinators Organization; NBNSC, National Board of Nutrition Support Certifications.

- Does he/she/they have strong family beliefs or influence from friends or other caregivers?
- Does he/she/they rely on Internet searches, and what types of websites do they currently review? Are he/she/they already selecting evidence-based resources or generic sites?
- Does he/she/they look to "social media influencers" for recommendations?
- Has he/she/they previously sought out working with an RD or non-AND credentialed "nutritionist"?

By dedicating time to ask such questions, providers can learn more about what is important to that specific patient and what things have or have not worked for them in the past. With this, providers can build a meaningful conversation and potentially

Table 2
Where to Find a Registered Dietitian
Academy of Nutrition & Dietetics   https://www.eatright.org/find-a-nutrition-expert

help the patient find new direction with evidence-based recommendations that are medically appropriate for their unique situation.

After gaining more information about a patient to customize the resources to be provided, it is important to consider the patient's literacy level. Some patients may be overwhelmed by the advanced language or complex sentences on handouts available from reliable resources. In this situation, it is helpful to provide handouts that are more picture based or ones that feature short, concise sentences. If creating your own materials for patients, it can be helpful to check the readability score available in a word processing program, and this can help ensure the materials are understandable for the patients' needs. Of note, the American Medical Association recommends a readability score at the sixth grade level or less for written materials.[22]

Along with choosing the most appropriate literacy level, it is important to understand which materials are available in different languages. If you do not have a material suitable for a patient's preferred language, it is important to see if the patient has another caregiver who can read a different language that you may have available in the written materials. In addition, if your practice is in a community that is rich in a specific language, it is beneficial to have native speakers review the content of the materials to make sure the translations will be well understood by both you the practitioner and the patient.

Finally, it is important to consider the format that will be best received by your patients. For some patients, having written materials will be the easiest to follow. Others may prefer digital copies of materials or the addresses of reliable websites they can return to on his/her/their own time. One consideration to make when providing written materials is the type of font being used. It is important to ensure the font is professional in appearance and easy to read. It is also beneficial to review the size of the font, as certain patients have specific visual needs. If selecting web pages or materials downloaded from the Internet, they may have the option to print in large fonts.

Selecting materials that take the patient's individual needs into consideration will make the education provided more personal and may help to increase a patient's receptiveness to the information. In addition, the customized materials may make it easier for patients to apply the recommendations into his/her/their daily life and increase the likelihood that the patient will succeed. For further assistance with disseminating nutrition education, it would be beneficial to make a referral for MNT provided by an RD who is trained to provide realistic and applicable education.

Cultural Considerations When Providing Education

When speaking with patients, it is important to consider their cultural and socioeconomic background in order to provide more meaningful nutrition education. Health inequities exist across the medical field. The term "cultural competence" was used in the past to describe the gold standard of care for patients with different backgrounds.[23] The Academy of Nutrition and Dietetics has moved away from this terminology, instead advocating for the practice of "cultural humility", defined as "...the ability to maintain an interpersonal stance that is other-oriented (or open to the other) in relation to the aspects of cultural identity that are most important to the person."[23] This in turn shifts the goal from attaining cultural competence toward a mindset of self-reflection in order to identify personal patterns of bias. As professionals, it is impera-tive to continue to seek opportunities to address personal biases to maximize the quality of patient care. In addition, it is important to be attentive to religious prefer-ences and home routines that may influence food choices. Examples of consider-ations to make when interviewing patients and providing education include the following:

- Cultural and religious food preferences
  - *Example:* Halal dietary guidelines, Kosher, Mormonism, Seventh Day Adventist
- Observed holidays that influence food choices
  - *Example:* Ash Wedneday, Good Friday, Passover, Ramadan, Yom Kippur, Lent
- Schedule/patient's typical pattern of food consumption
  - *Example:* Number of meals eaten per day, work schedule
- Home environment for shopping/cooking
  - *Example:* Who in the home completes these tasks? What facilities does the pa-tient have for cooking (eg, a hot plate vs a full kitchen; a functioning refriger-ator/freezer; storage space)? What foods are available at neighborhood stores? How are they able to transport food back to the home?
- Use of Government Assistance Programs
  - *Example:* Supplemental Nutrition Assistance Program (SNAP), Special Supple-mental Nutrition Women Infants and Children (WIC).

Language Considerations

Patients, families, and caregivers may speak different languages or have specific di-alects they prefer to use to communicate that differ from that of his/her/their care pro-vider. Despite efforts to communicate with patients who have culturally diverse backgrounds, some health information may be lost in translation. Of note, the Afford-able Care Act (section 1557) protects individuals with Limited English Proficiency (LEP) by requiring providers who participate in federally funded programs and activities to provide free, accurate, and timely interpreter services.[24] With this, an interpreter must be used when there is a language discrepancy between patient and provider.[25] In a descriptive commentary aiming to improve communication in the health care setting, Hadziabdic and Hjelm[26] review the negative patient impact of not using an interpreter in the health care setting. Specifically, "...patients reported fewer symp-toms, particularly mental ones, and that important aspects such as wound care, foot care, dietary advice and experience of pain were documented to a lower extent."[26] When choosing an interpreter, these investigators[26] also note that it is important to involve the patient and their family to decide the type (trained, family, bilingual provider) and mode (face to face or telephone) to select the best individual to facilitate the session. Regional dialects (especially for larger languages) and diverse ethnicities within language groups may also influence the interpretation of the individ-ual conducting the interview.[25,26] Preparing for and identifying the appropriate inter-preter will minimize the risk of inaccurate translations due to differing regional dialects between the patient and the interpreter.[26] Establishing preferred methods of communication can help providers improve both patient and provider satisfaction, while better meeting a patient's needs.[27]

Of note, ambulatory care settings may have a contract with a language line or in-person interpreter service. If available, it is best practice for providers to use these ser-vices to facilitate information delivery to their patients, families, and caregivers. If a site does not have access to these services, it would be helpful to confirm preferred

Table 3
Lingual services available for providers

Service	Website
Language Line	https://www.languageline.com/s/Healthcare
Lion Bridge	https://www.lionbridge.com/content-transformation-services/interpretation-services
Alta	https://www.altalang.com/get-started/interpretation
Deaf Interpreter Services	https://www.deaf-interpreter.com/
Community Interpreter Services	https://communityinterpreterservices.org/

language ahead of a patient's visit in order to make appropriate communication and resource arrangements. Use of both interpreter services and provision of language concordant patient education materials can lead to improved health care delivery.[27] **Table 3** provides examples of culturally diverse lingual services that may be beneficial if a primary care site is not already contracted with an appropriate company.

Disease-Specific Patient Resources

Appropriate selection of patient education resources requires health care providers to consider the disease state being treated. Modern day access to Internet search engines has resulted in both several solutions, as well as several challenges, for health care providers. Approximately 1 in 3 US adults report turning to online resources in hopes of self-identifying a medical diagnosis or to obtain additional information regarding a health-related complaint.[28] In addition, the data collected from the Health Information National Trends Survey (HINTS 5, cycle 2) was used to generate population estimates that suggest 70.14% of US adults digitally seek health information.[29] UK-based researchers also found that the number of people reporting that they have used online resources for health information increased from 37% in 2005 to 69% in 2013.[30] Health information seekers are often left to their own devices to evaluate the credibility and reliability of sources they have encountered online, with research informing us that low health literacy can increase their vulnerability to falling victim to the sea of misinformation throughout the Internet.[31] Thus, it is necessary for health care professionals to direct patients toward credible and reliable online resources. Federal Government agencies, large professional organizations, and respected medical schools often provide evidence-based disease-specific nutrition resources. Examples of credible sources are provided later. Most websites provide information that is easily printable in web page or PDF formats.

The *American Cancer Society*[32] Web site covers oncological nutrition topics ranging from cancer prevention, healthy recipes, advice for eating out, and information on nutritional management of treatment-related side effects (loss of appetite, diarrhea, taste changes, mouth sores, and so forth). This website can be translated into 12 different languages.

The *American Diabetes Association (ADA)*[33] website provides patients and providers with a *Patient Education Library* allowing access to a variety of printable nutrition-related handouts centered around diabetes care and management available in 10 different languages. The *Diabetes Food Hub* is also accessible via the ADA Web site and contains recipe and meal ideas including a "Budget-Friendly" section. Please note the *Diabetes Food Hub* is only available in English, although the online shop has print recipe books available for purchase in Spanish.

The *Association of Diabetes Care and Education Specialists*[34] website has resources for patients that include nutrition-focused learning materials and how to connect to diabetes care and education specialists or diabetes education programs. Online materials are available in several languages.

The *American Heart Association*[35] website contains several articles and infographics related to nutritional prevention and management of cardiovascular diseases, which are available in English and Spanish.

The *Centers for Disease Control and Prevention*[36] website provides access to extensive array nutritional information specific to a variety of disease states including cancer, diabetes, chronic obstructive pulmonary disease, heart disease, weight management, chronic kidney disease, stroke, and traumatic brain injury. Nutrition-related health information is available in English and Spanish.

At the *National Institutes of Health (NIH)*[37] website, specific institutes such as the *National Cancer Institute*[38] and the *National Institute of Diabetes and Digestive and Kidney Diseases*[39] serve as excellent sources of credible information about disease-specific nutrition management. Web site information and translation is available in English and Spanish languages.

The *NYC Health*[40] website provides translation of the entire site into 100+ languages and, although NYC-based, is not only specific to those practicing or residing in the metro NYC area. Nutrition information is available on several disease-specific topics including diabetes and cancer. Information is also available for pregnancy and gestational diabetes, as well as general healthful nutrition guidance, which includes culturally appropriate and multilingual versions of the MyPlate[41] educational tool. Education resources are available in 10+ languages.

Please note that some web pages, such as NYC Health,[40] allow for translation of the entire website in several languages, whereas others only provide select printable materials in alternative languages. In many cases, such as with the NIH,[37] site-wide languages are limited to English and Spanish. Health care providers should familiarize themselves with the aforementioned resources to best serve their patients' needs. An overview of credible, disease-specific resources and language availability can be found in **Table 4**.

Nutrition education materials are updated on a continuous basis, as new scientific literature dictates best practices. A working relationship with an RD offers physicians and other health care providers access to a reliable expert in the field with up-to-date information on practice guidelines and tools.

RESOURCES FOR PROVIDERS
Nutrition Resources

Patients, family, and caregivers often turn to physicians as a resource for nutrition recommendations; however, the nutrition education physicians receive in medical school is scant. Adams, Butsch, and Kohlmeier[42] conducted a survey on the extent and type of nutrition education provided in medical schools compared with recommended targets. Of the 121 responding medical schools, the reported average required time spent on nutrition education was 19 hours instead of the recommended 25 hours with most nutrition education taking place in preclinical training. As a result, "...many physicians do not feel confident in their clinical nutrition skills, particularly when it comes to dealing with overweight or obese patients."[42] The following resources provide credible nutrition information intended for the medical community to enhance and guide clinical practice.

The *Academy of Nutrition and Dietetics*[43] is the largest organization of nutrition professionals in all settings. The Academy provides position papers, expert testimony at

Table 4
Disease-specific Online Resources

Online Resource	Language Availability	Website
American Cancer Society	English Spanish Arabic Chinese French Haitian Creole Hindi Korean Polish Portuguese Russian Tagalog Vietnamese	https://www.cancer.org
American Diabetes Association	English Spanish Arabic Chinese French Haitian Creole Korean Portuguese Russian Tagalog Vietnamese	https://www.diabetes.org
Association of Diabetes Care and Education Specialists	English Spanish Chinese French Tagalog	https://www.diabeteseducator.org
American Heart Association	English Spanish	https://www.heart.org
Centers for Disease Control and Prevention	English Spanish	https://www.cdc.gov
National Institutes of Health	English Spanish	https://www.nih.gov NIDDK: https://www.niddk.nih.gov NCI: https://www.cancer.gov
NYC Health	English Spanish Arabic Bengali Chinese French Haitian Creole Italian Korean Polish Russian Urdu Yiddish	https://www1.nyc.gov MyPlate Resources: https://www1.nyc.gov/site/doh/health/ health-topics/eating-well.page

hearings, and comments on public policy. It publishes the Journal of the Academy of Nutrition and Dietetics and oversees the Evidence Analysis Library. On the website, https://www.eatright.org, a variety of available webinars, textbooks, clinical resources, and education materials are available for purchase. In addition, there are multiple articles that can be useful for patients. Topics include food, health and lifestyle, and fitness.

- The *Evidence Analysis Library*[44] consists of nutrition guidelines graded for strength of evidence.
- The *Journal of the Academy of Nutrition and Dietetics*[45] is a monthly peer-reviewed journal. There is original research on multiple topics such as health and disease, dietary habits and interventions, medical nutrition therapy, food service, management, nutrigenomics, and epidemiology.

The *Commission on Dietetic Registration*[6] is the credentialing agency of the Academy of Nutrition and Dietetics. It upholds the standards for maintaining certification and the code of ethics for Dietitians, diet technicians, and all board specialty certifications. Here, there is more information on the process of becoming an RD or obtaining a specialty board certification and the code of ethics for the profession.

The *American Society for Parenteral and Enteral Nutrition (ASPEN)*[46] is an interdisciplinary organization that includes RDs, nurses, pharmacists, physicians, scientists, students, and other allied health professionals in clinical practice of nutrition support. Sources for information on parenteral nutrition (PN) and enteral nutrition (EN) can be found on their website. There are also clinical care guidelines and resources, including academic journals, information about malnutrition, and resources for specific patient populations or health care management. ASPEN releases 2 journals, the Journal of Parenteral and Enteral Nutrition and Nutrition in Clinical Practice.[47]

The *American Society for Nutrition*[48] is an organization with the goal of advancing the science, education, and practice of nutrition. They advocate for nutrition research and the science of nutrition. The organization publishes the Journal of Nutrition, The American Journal of Clinical Nutrition, Advances in Nutrition, and Current Developments in Nutrition. They also educate policymakers to provide recommendations for science-based policies. Through the website you can access a variety of webinars and an online learning portal with valuable materials for clinicians.

UpToDate[49] is a collection of clinical reviews with evidence-graded recommendations under continuous review, presented with the aim of aiding with real-time clinical decision-making, and includes extensive and easily searchable nutrition content.

The *Oley Foundation*[50] is a nonprofit organization for patients who receive home EN or PN support. The website includes multiple resources and articles that address a variety of topics such as EN basics, tube feed troubleshooting, nutrition support weaning, choosing a home care agency, patient stories and more, useful for clinicians, patients, and family members.

Insurance Coverage and Nutrition Support Resources

There are numerous components to consider when preparing a patient to receive home EN or PN support. It is important to note that infusion companies can provide both EN and PN support, whereas traditional pharmacies are not typically able to provide these services. Traditional pharmacies can be limited by multiple authorization requirements, lack of stock of EN formulas and supplies, and the inability to compound

Table 5
Overview of nutrition support Medicare coverage and criteria

Type of Nutrition Support	Medicare Coverage	Criteria
Enteral Nutrition	Medicare Part B or Prosthetic Device Coverage may cover the formula and all medical supplies required	"A patient with a functioning gastrointestinal tract who, due to pathology to, or non-function of, the structures that normally permit food to reach the digestive tract, cannot maintain weight and strength commensurate with his or her general condition.[49]" Sole Source of Nutrition Long Term, generally accepted as ≥3 months Common Diagnoses: Severe Dysphagia or obstructing masses in the upper GI tract
Parenteral Nutrition	Medicare Part B may cover the parenteral formula and medical supplies required for provision Medicare Part D Drug plan may cover the parenteral formula	"...severe pathology of the alimentary tract which does not allow absorption of sufficient nutrients to maintain weight and strength commensurate with the patient's general condition.[49]" Long Term, generally accepted as ≥3 months

PN. Durable medical equipment providers typically carry enteral formulas and necessary supplies to provide EN.

Insurance coverage for nutrition support varies by payer. Many insurance providers require preauthorization or authorization for coverage and will typically require a prescription, along with documentation supporting the coverage criteria.

It is important for providers to prescribe clinically appropriate, targeted, safe, and cost-effective regimens. It is also important for providers to assess the patient's ability to afford the prescribed regimen if the patient does not have a primary or secondary insurance that will cover nutrition support. Of note, some insurance companies may not cover the cost of enteral formula, given the expectation that the cost of formula is replacing the cost of groceries. Although this may be true for standard formulas, the cost of hydrolyzed or metabolic formulas can be several hundred dollars per month. Some states, including New York State, have mandates that require insurance coverage of medical foods if prescribed by a physician. Coverage varies for oral supplements, and stringent criteria often apply. Enteral supplies, including syringes, gravity bags, or enteral pumps, are typically covered by insurance companies; however, some will not cover an enteral pump unless the patient does not tolerate bolus or gravity feeds. Although detailing all insurance coverage is outside the scope of this article, a brief summary of the coverage provided by Medicare,[51] which has some of the strictest criteria, is available in **Table 5**.

To ensure all the patient's needs are being addressed, the infusion company selected should have a multidisciplinary team including pharmacists, nurses, and Dietitians. Companies with educational programs and resources can help the patient feel more comfortable and confident managing these therapies at home. Using an infusion company with a nationwide presence will allow the patient to travel while still receiving their needed nutrition support.

SUMMARY

RDs complete extensive training to provide individualized nutrition education and care; however, all health care practitioners share the responsibility of disseminating nutrition information to patients in order to prevent health misinformation. Effective nutrition education includes taking a patient's readiness to learn, literacy level, culture, language, and specific disease state into consideration. As a provider, it is vital to engage in meaningful discussions while sharing appropriate resources to help patients achieve his/her/their goals and make realistic changes.

DISCLOSURE

M. Christensen is employed by Coram CVS Specialty Infusion Services (Coram). All other authors have no conflicts of interest or funding to disclose.

REFERENCES

1. What is a Registered Dietitian Nutritionist. EatRightPro. 2021. Available at: https://www.eatrightpro.org/about-us/what-is-an-rdn-and-dtr/what-is-a-registered-dietitian-nutritionist. Accessed November 13, 2021.
2. MNT versus nutrition education. EatRightPro. 2006. Available at: https://www.eatrightpro.org/payment/coding-and-billing/mnt-vs-nutrition-education. Accessed November 13, 2021.
3. Every registered dietitian is a nutritionist, but not every nutritionist is a registered dietitian. EatRightPro. 2021. Available at: https://www.eatrightpro.org/about-us/what-is-an-rdn-and-dtr/what-is-a-registered-dietitian-nutritionist/every-registered-dietitian-is-a-nutritionist-but-not-every-nutritionist-is-a-registered-dietitian. Accessed November 13, 2021.
4. FAQs about careers in dietetics. EatRightPro. 2020. Available at: https://www.eatrightpro.org/acend/students-and-advancing-education/information-for-students/faqs-about-careers-in-dietetics. Accessed November 13, 2021.
5. Registered dietitian nutritionist fact sheet. EatRightPro. 2020. Available at: https://www.eatrightpro.org/acend/students-and-advancing-education/information-for-students/registered-dietitian-nutritionist-fact-sheet. Accessed November 13, 2021.
6. About CDR. CDRnet. 2021. Available at: https://www.cdrnet.org/about. Accessed November 13, 2021.
7. Licensure and professional regulation of dietitians. EatRightPro. 2021. Available at: https://www.eatrightpro.org/advocacy/licensure/professional-regulation-of-dietitians. Accessed November 13, 2021.
8. Andersen D, Baird S, Bates T, et al. Academy of Nutrition and Dietetics: Revised 2017 standards of practice in nutrition care and standards of professional performance for registered dietitian nutritionists. J Acad Nutr Diet 2017;118(1): 132–40.e15. https://doi.org/10.1016/j.jand.2017.10.003.
9. Code of ethics for the profession. Code of Ethics for the Nutrition and Dietetics Profession. Available at: https://www.eatrightpro.org/-/media/eatrightpro-files/career/code-of-ethics/coeforthenutritionanddieteticsprofession.pdf?

la=en&hash=0C9D1622C51782F12A0D6004A28CDAC0CE99A032. Accessed November 13, 2021.
10. Peregrin T. Revisions to the code of ethics for the nutrition and Dietetics Profession. J Acad Nutr Diet 2018;118(9):1764–7. https://doi.org/10.1016/j.jand.2018.05.028.
11. Referring patients to an RDN. EatRightPro. 2021. Available at: https://www.eatrightpro.org/about-us/what-is-an-rdn-and-dtr/work-with-an-rdn-or-dtr/referring-patients-to-an-rdn. Accessed November 13, 2021.
12. Advanced Practitioner Certification in Clinical Nutrition. Available at: https://www.cdrnet.org/board-certification-in-advanced-practice. Accessed November 22, 2021.
13. The Academy of Lactation Policy and Practice. The CLC - Certified Lactation Counselor. 2021. Available at: https://alpp.org/certifications/certifications-clc. Accessed November 22, 2021.
14. Apply for the CDCES credential. CDCES. 2021. Available at: https://www.cbdce.org/become-certified. Accessed November 22, 2021.
15. Certification Overview. International Association of Eating Disorders. 2021. Professionals Foundation Available at: http://www.iaedp.com/certification-overview/. Accessed November 22, 2021.
16. Board Certified Specialist Home. Certifications: Board Certified Specialist - Commission on Dietetics Registration. 2021. Available at: https://www.cdrnet.org/certifications/board-certified-specialist. Accessed November 22, 2021.
17. Specialty Practice Experience. Specialty Practice Experience - Commission on Dietetics Registration. 2021. Available at: https://www.cdrnet.org/certifications/specialty-practice-experience. Accessed November 22, 2021.
18. International Board of Lactation Consultant Examiners. IBLCE. 2021. Available at: https://iblce.org/. Accessed November 22, 2021.
19. Page Certification Main. NBNSC. 2021. Available at: https://www.nutritioncare.org/NBNSC/Certification/Certification_Main_Page/. Accessed November 22, 2021.
20. Certified clinical transplant dietitian. NATCO. Available at: https://www.natco1.org/certifications/cctd/. Accessed November 22, 2021.
21. Find a Nutrition Expert. EatRight. 2021. Available at: https://www.eatright.org/find-a-nutrition-expert. Accessed November 28, 2021.
22. Weis BD. Health literacy: a Manual for clinicians. Chicago: American Medical Association, American Medical Foundation; 2003.
23. Lund A, Latortue KY, Rodriguez J. Dietetic training: Understanding racial inequity in power and privilege. J Acad Nutr Diet 2021;121(8):1437–40. https://doi.org/10.1016/j.jand.2020.09.041.
24. Office for Civil Rights. Section 1557 of the Patient Protection and Affordable Care Act. HHS.gov. 2021. https://www.hhs.gov/civil-rights/for-individuals/section-1557/index.html. Accessed February 24, 2022.
25. World Medical Association. Medical ethics Manual. In: Ferney-voltaire. 3rd edition. France: World Medical Association; 2015. p. 43–53.
26. Hadziabdic E, Hjelm K. Working with interpreters: Practical advice for use of an interpreter in Healthcare. Int J Evidence-Based Healthc 2013;11(1):69–76. https://doi.org/10.1111/1744-1609.12005.
27. Al Shamsi H, Almutairi AG, Al Mashrafi S, et al. Implications of language barriers for Healthcare: A systematic review. Oman Med J 2020;35(2). https://doi.org/10.5001/omj.2020.40.

28. Fox S, Duggan M. Health Online 2013. Pew Research Center. 2013. Available at: https://www.pewresearch.org/internet/2013/01/15/health-online-2013/.
29. Ratcliff CL, Krakow M, Greenberg-Worisek A, et al. Digital Health engagement in the US population: Insights from the 2018 Health Information National Trends Survey. Am J Public Health 2021;111(7):1348–51. https://doi.org/10.2105/ajph.2021.306282.
30. Dutton W, Blank G. Worldinternetproject. 2013. Cultures of the Internet: The Internet in Britain. Available at: http://www.worldinternetproject.net/_files/_Published/23/820_oxis2011_report.pdf.
31. Diviani N, van den Putte B, Giani S, et al. Low health literacy and evaluation of online health information: A systematic review of the literature. J Med Internet Res 2015;17(5). https://doi.org/10.2196/jmir.4018.
32. Information and resources about cancer: Breast, colon, lung, prostate, skin. American Cancer Society. 2021. Available at: https://www.cancer.org/. Accessed November 20, 2021.
33. Home. American Diabetes Association | Research, Education, Advocacy. 2021. Available at: https://www.diabetes.org/. Accessed November 20, 2021.
34. Association Home. of diabetes care & education specialists. 2021. Available at: https://www.diabeteseducator.org/home. Accessed November 20, 2021.
35. American Heart Association. 2021. Available at: www.heart.org; https://www.heart.org/. Accessed November 20, 2021.
36. Centers for Disease Control and Prevention. 2021. Available at: https://www.cdc.gov/. Accessed November 20, 2021.
37. National Institutes of Health. 2021. Available at: https://www.nih.gov/. Accessed November 20, 2021.
38. Comprehensive Cancer Information. National Cancer Institute. 2021. Available at: https://www.cancer.gov/. Accessed November 29, 2021.
39. National Institute of Diabetes and digestive and kidney diseases (NIDDK). National Institute of Diabetes and Digestive and Kidney Diseases. 2021. Available at: https://www.niddk.nih.gov/. Accessed November 20, 2021.
40. NYC Health. 2021. Available at: https://www1.nyc.gov/site/doh/index.page. Accessed November 20, 2021.
41. Nutrition Tips. Nutrition Tips - NYC Health. 2021. Available at: https://www1.nyc.gov/site/doh/health/health-topics/eating-well.page. Accessed November 20, 2021.
42. Adams KM, Butsch WS, Kohlmeier M. The State of Nutrition Education at US Medical Schools. J Biomed Education 2015;2015:1–7. https://doi.org/10.1155/2015/357627.
43. Academy of Nutrition and Dietetics. EatRight. Available at: https://www.eatright.org/. Accessed November 20, 2021.
44. Welcome to the Evidence Analysis Library. your Food and Nutrition Research Resource. EAL. Available at: https://www.andeal.org/. Accessed November 20, 2021.
45. Journal of The American Dietetics Association. Available at: https://www.jandonline.org/. Accessed November 20, 2021.
46. American Society for Parenteral and Enteral Nutrition (ASPEN). American Society for enteral and parenteral nutrition. ASPEN. 2022. https://www.nutritioncare.org/. Accessed November 20, 2021.
47. Journals. ASPEN | Journals. Available at: https://www.nutritioncare.org/Publications/Journals/. Accessed November 20, 2021.

48. American Society for Nutrition. 2020. Available at: https://nutrition.org/. Accessed November 20, 2021.
49. Uptodate. Evidence-based clinical decision support. 2021. Available at: https://www.wolterskluwer.com/en/solutions/uptodate. Accessed November 20, 2021.
50. Oley Foundation. 2021. Available at: https://oley.org/. Accessed November 20, 2021.
51. Determination Enteral and Parenteral Nutrition Therapy. CMS. Available at: https://www.cms.gov/medicare-coverage-database/view/ncd.aspx? NCDId =242&ver=1. Accessed November 22, 2021.

Moving?

Make sure your subscription moves with you!

To notify us of your new address, find your **Clinics Account Number** (located on your mailing label above your name), and contact customer service at:

Email: journalscustomerservice-usa@elsevier.com

800-654-2452 (subscribers in the U.S. & Canada)
314-447-8871 (subscribers outside of the U.S. & Canada)

Fax number: 314-447-8029

**Elsevier Health Sciences Division
Subscription Customer Service
3251 Riverport Lane
Maryland Heights, MO 63043**

*To ensure uninterrupted delivery of your subscription, please notify us at least 4 weeks in advance of move.

Printed and bound by CPI Group (UK) Ltd, Croydon, CR0 4YY

03/10/2024

01040466-0019